CANCER ETIOLOGY, DIAGNOSIS AND TREATMENTS

CODING FOR DISEASE

GENES AND CANCER

CANCER ETIOLOGY, DIAGNOSIS AND TREATMENTS

Additional books in this series can be found on Nova's website under the Series tab.

Additional e-books in this series can be found on Nova's website under the e-book tab.

GENETICS - RESEARCH AND ISSUES

Additional books in this series can be found on Nova's website under the Series tab.

Additional e-books in this series can be found on Nova's website under the e-book tab.

CANCER ETIOLOGY, DIAGNOSIS AND TREATMENTS

CODING FOR DISEASE GENES AND CANCER

MARC LACROIX

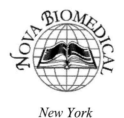

New York

Copyright © 2013 by Nova Science Publishers, Inc.

All rights reserved. No part of this book may be reproduced, stored in a retrieval system or transmitted in any form or by any means: electronic, electrostatic, magnetic, tape, mechanical photocopying, recording or otherwise without the written permission of the Publisher.

For permission to use material from this book please contact us:
Telephone 631-231-7269; Fax 631-231-8175
Web Site: http://www.novapublishers.com

NOTICE TO THE READER

The Publisher has taken reasonable care in the preparation of this book, but makes no expressed or implied warranty of any kind and assumes no responsibility for any errors or omissions. No liability is assumed for incidental or consequential damages in connection with or arising out of information contained in this book. The Publisher shall not be liable for any special, consequential, or exemplary damages resulting, in whole or in part, from the readers' use of, or reliance upon, this material. Any parts of this book based on government reports are so indicated and copyright is claimed for those parts to the extent applicable to compilations of such works.

Independent verification should be sought for any data, advice or recommendations contained in this book. In addition, no responsibility is assumed by the publisher for any injury and/or damage to persons or property arising from any methods, products, instructions, ideas or otherwise contained in this publication.

This publication is designed to provide accurate and authoritative information with regard to the subject matter covered herein. It is sold with the clear understanding that the Publisher is not engaged in rendering legal or any other professional services. If legal or any other expert assistance is required, the services of a competent person should be sought. FROM A DECLARATION OF PARTICIPANTS JOINTLY ADOPTED BY A COMMITTEE OF THE AMERICAN BAR ASSOCIATION AND A COMMITTEE OF PUBLISHERS.

Additional color graphics may be available in the e-book version of this book.

Library of Congress Cataloging-in-Publication Data

ISBN: 978-1-62257-817-7

Library of Congress Control Number: 2013937386

Published by Nova Science Publishers, Inc. † New York

This book is dedicated to Anne-Marie Corman (1934 – 2011)

Contents

Preface		ix
Chapter 1	A Detailed List of Major Cancer Genes	1
Chapter 2	Gene Fusions in Cancer	75
Chapter 3	Gene Amplification in Cancer	97
Chapter 4	Low Penetrance Sites in Cancer: Candidate Genes	115
Chapter 5	Familial Cancer Syndromes	135
Chapter 6	Epigenetics and Cancer	167
Abbreviations		181
Index		183

Preface

Our knowledge on the genetic basis of cancer developed slowly from the end of the 19th century onwards. More precisely, since David von Hansemann and Theodor Boveri found an association between aberrant mitoses and malignant tumors. However, the existence of "cancer families" had been suspected centuries ago. Most data linking genes and cancer have been accumulated in the last forty years. Cancer is now recognized as being essentially a disease caused by mutation, or altered expression, of genes.

Cancer is characterized by uncontrolled cell division and the potential of the cells to invade surrounding tissues and spread around the body. These changes in cellular behavior are the result of alterations in the function or levels of the proteins that control these processes. And these alterations are, in turn, usually caused by mutations, or changes in expression, of the genes encoding the proteins.

There has been considerable progress in identifying the genes and their mutations involved in both sporadic and familial cancers. In addition, it has been recognized that as well as genetic mutations, epigenetic changes play an important role in the development of cancer.

Of the estimated 30,000 genes in the human genome, currently more than 250 are known to play a role in the development of cancer. A number of these genes are described in chapter 1: *"A detailed list of major cancer genes"*.

Various types of genetic alterations can occur; some of the more common types are missense point mutation, nonsense point mutation, frameshift mutation, and the "chromosomal mutations": inversion, deletion, translocation, amplification. Chromosomal mutations may sometimes generate gene fusions and the production of hybrid transcripts (see chapter 2: *"Gene fusions in cancer"*). The role of gene amplification in the development of cancer has also been demonstrated (see chapter 3: *"Gene amplification in cancer"*)

During the last years, attention has largely shifted from the identification of rare high-risk genetic mutations to a hunt for lower risk gene polymorphisms, many of which are likely to be common within the population (see chapter 4: *"Low penetrance sites in cancer : candidate genes"*). The challenge is to identify these polymorphisms and to find strategies to reduce the risk of them contributing to cancer development.

While a majority of cancers are sporadic, some cases of cancer are caused by the inheritance of a high-risk mutation in a particular gene (see chapter 5: *"Familial cancer syndromes"*). It is estimated that around one per cent of all cancers are caused by these high-risk mutations, which generally affect tumor suppressor genes. Some high-risk susceptibility genes are associated with very rare familial cancer syndromes. These are usually characterized by a range of cancers occurring at different, often unusual, sites. Despite the rarity of these syndromes, the large numbers of cases in some affected families have helped in identifying the faulty genes involved. Other high-risk, inherited mutations have been identified that predispose to some of the more common cancers, including breast, ovarian and bowel cancer. People carrying these mutations are at high risk of developing the associated cancer(s), but overall the mutations are responsible for only a small proportion of all cases of the cancer.

Epigenetics is the study of mechanisms that alter gene expression and activity, without involving changes in genetic sequence. The best studied of these mechanisms are biochemical modifications, including changes in methylation of CpG dinucleotides and changes in histone acetylation or methylation (see chapter 6: *Epigenetics and cancer*). The normal pattern of epigenetic modifications in cells, the epigenome, arises during embryogenesis and development, and is inherited by daughter cells after mitosis of differentiated cells. However, temporary, reversible changes in epigenetic modification are essential for changes in chromosomal structure to allow, for example, transcription or DNA replication. But, some abnormal or prolonged changes to the epigenome can contribute to the development of cancer.

***

Born in 1963 in Verviers (Wallonia, Belgium), Marc Lacroix has been working for more than 20 years in several academic institutions (University of Liège, Free University of Brussels and Jules Bordet Institute). He is now at InTextoResearch (ITR@iname.com, Baelen, Belgium), an agency devoted to scientific information on cancer.

Chapter 1

A Detailed List of Major Cancer Genes

Abstract

The fact that cancer may result from alterations in specific genes has been documented for decades. Recent technological advances in genome analysis and intense research in the field have allowed to conclude that alterations in only a few dozens genes are of prime importance in causing or aggravating cancer. These genes, as well as their common alterations, are presented here.

Introduction

Decades ago, it was shown that mutations in genes can cause cancer. Some genes ("proto-oncogenes") may be activated by mutation to oncogenes, which trigger cancer; others ("tumor suppressors") may lose their function upon alteration.

Years of subsequent research have led to the general acceptance of the paradigm that sequential accumulation of genetic errors or mutations in proto-oncogenes and tumor suppressors eventually transforms a normal cell into a tumor cell (Vogelstein and Kinzler 2004). It is now clear that, while more than 30,000 coding genes have been identified in humans, only a very limited subset of these may play a causative or aggravating role in cancer.

For instance, an analysis of 13,023 genes in 11 breast and 11 colorectal cancers revealed that individual tumors could accumulate an average of approximately 90 mutant genes, with only a subset of these contributing to the neoplastic process (Sjöblom et al. 2006). Some genes are frequently altered, in many tumor types: this is notably the case for TP53 and CDKN2A.

Some genes are altered mainly in specific tumor types, as observed i.e. for RET and thyroid cancer, or PHOX2B and CNS tumors. This chapter aims to present about one hundred genes involved in cancer.

Cancer Genes

ABL1 (9q34.1)
V-Abl Abelson Murine Leukemia Viral Oncogene Homolog 1

Function
ABL1 (De Braekeleer et al. 2011) encodes a protein tyrosine kinase involved in cell differentiation, division, and adhesion, and in stress response. It interacts with a large variety of cellular proteins including signaling adaptors, kinases, phosphatases, cell cycle regulators, transcription factors and cytoskeletal proteins. Activity of ABL1 protein is negatively regulated by its SH3 domain, and deletion of the SH3 domain turns ABL1 into an oncogene.

Cancer-Related Gene Alterations
- An ins(22;9)(q11;q34q34), leading to BCR-ABL1 fusion gene, is observed in chronic myeloid leukemia (CML).
- A t(9;22)(q34;q11) (BCR-ABL1) is a cause of CML. In fact, all CML patients have a t(9;22), at least at the molecular level. A similar translocation is found in acute myeloid leukemia (AML) and in acute lymphoblastic leukemia (ALL).
- In ALL, another translocation, t(9;12)(q34;p12) (ETV6-ABL1), may occasionally occur.
- In T-cell ALL ("T-ALL"), t(9;9)(q34;q34) (NUP214-ABL1) and t(9;14)(q34;q32) (EML1-ABL1) are also observed. The NUP214-ABL1 gene is the second most prevalent fusion gene involving ABL1 in malignant hemopathies.
- In B-cell ALL ("B-ALL") t(1;9)(q24;q34) (RCSD1-ABL1), t(1;9)(p34;q34) (SFPQ-ABL1) and t(9;10)(q34;q22.3) (ZMIZ1-ABL1) are also observed.
- Somatic ABL1 mutations have been observed mainly in hematopoietic and lymphoid tissue cancers (up to 30% of cases). They are substitutions, exclusively, and most of them are found in a region (corresponding to amino acids 232-499) associated to protein kinase activity.

AKT1 (14q32.32-q32.33)
RAC-Alpha Serine/Threonine-Protein Kinase

Function
AKT1 (Heron-Milhavet et al. 2011) encodes one of 3 closely related serine/threonine protein kinases (AKT1, AKT2 and AKT3) which regulate many processes including metabolism, proliferation, cell survival, growth and angiogenesis. AKT1-specific substrates have been recently identified, including palladin, which phosphorylation modulates cytoskeletal organization and cell motility; prohibitin, playing an important role in cell metabolism and proliferation; and cyclin-dependent kinase inhibitor 1 (better known as p21 / WAF1), for which phosphorylation at residue 'threonine-145' induces its release from CDK2 and its cytoplasmic relocalization. These recent findings indicate that among AKT proteins, the AKT1 isoform has a more specific role in cell motility and proliferation.

Cancer-Related Gene Alterations
- AKT1 somatic point mutations have been identified mainly in breast, colorectal and ovarian cancers. Mutations have also been found in urinary tract, thyroid, endometrial and prostate cancers. More than 99% of these somatic mutations are substitutions. Most mutations are found in a region coding for the first 50 amino acids ("pleckstrin homology" domain), with a mutation hotspot at amino acid 17.

AKT2 (19q13.1-q13.2)
V-Akt Murine Thymoma Viral Oncogene Homolog 2

Function

AKT2 (Heron-Milhavet et al. 2011) encodes one of 3 closely related serine/threonine protein kinases (AKT1, AKT2 and AKT3) which regulate many processes including metabolism, proliferation, cell survival, growth and angiogenesis. One specific AKT2 substrate identified recently is PITX2. Phosphorylation of PITX2 impairs its association with the CCND1 (encoding cyclin D1) mRNA-stabilizing complex thus shortening the half-life of cyclin D1. AKT2 seems also to be the principal isoform responsible of the regulation of glucose uptake by cells. AKT2 is a putative oncogene.

Cancer-Related Gene Alterations
- Various AKT2 somatic point mutations have been identified in breast, colorectal and lung cancers; more than 80% of these somatic mutations are substitutions and are found in the N-terminal "pleckstrin homology" domain of AKT2.
- AKT2 amplification and overexpression have been observed in ovarian tumors and ovarian cancer cell lines.

ALK (2p23)
Anaplastic Lymphoma Receptor Tyrosine Kinase

Function

ALK (Yauch and Settleman 2012) encodes a tyrosine kinase receptor of the insulin receptor superfamily. It is a dependence receptor, which may exert antagonist functions, proapoptotic or antiapoptotic, depending on the absence or presence of a ligand. Most ALK mutations affect the tyrosine kinase domain.

Cancer-Related Gene Alterations
- ALK is involved in numerous translocations and subsequent gene fusions:
    - (ALCL);
    - inv(2)(p23q35) with ATIC is associated to ALCL and inflammatory myofibroblastic tumor (IMT);
    - t(2;11)(p23;p15) with CARS is associated to IMT;
    - t(2;17)(p23;q23) with CLTC is associated to IMT and non-Hodgkin lymphoma (NHL);

- t(2;22)(p23;q11.2) with CLTCL1 is associated to NHL;
- inv(2)(p21p23) with EML4 is associated to non-small cells lung cancer (NSCLC);
- t(X;2)(q11;p23) with MSN is associated to ALCL;
- t(2;22)(p23;q11.2-q12) with MYH9 is associated to NHL;
- t(2;5)(p23;q35) with NPM1 is associated to NHL and IMT;
- t(2;2)(p23;q11-q13) with RANBP2 is associated to IMT;
- t(2;17)(p23;q25) with RNF213 is associated to NHL;
- t(2;4)(p23;q21) with SEC31A is associated to IMT;
- t(2;3)(p23;q21) with TFG is associated to NHL, NSCLC, ALCL;
- inv(2)(p23;q11-13) and t(1;2)(q25;p23) with TPM3, are associated to IMT and ALCL;
- t(2;19)(p23;p13.1) with TPM4 is associated to NHL, IMT, and squamous cell carcinoma (SCC).

In a great majority of cases, abnormal proteins are made of the N-term amino acids from the partner gene fused to the 563 C-term amino acids from ALK (i.e. the entire cytoplasmic portion of ALK with the tyrosine kinase domain). The partner gene seems to provoke the dimerization of the fused X-ALK, which should lead to constitutive autophosphorylation and activation of the ALK tyrosine kinase.

- Germline and somatic mutations or gene amplification of ALK may cause familial and sporadic neuroblastoma, respectively. Various point mutations have been described, with two hotspots corresponding to amino acids F1174 and R1275. The most frequent germline mutations in familial cases are G1128A, R1192P and R1275Q. The most frequent somatic mutations in sporadic cases are F1174L/I and F1245C/V.

APC (5q21-q22)
Adenomatous Polyposis Coli

Function
APC (Minde et al. 2011) encodes a tumor suppressor protein that indirectly regulates transcription of a number of critical cell proliferation genes, through its interaction with the transcription factor β-catenin (encoded by CTNNB1 gene). APC is also involved in cell adhesion and migration, and in cell apoptosis.

Cancer-Related Gene Alterations
- Germline mutations of APC cause a spectrum of diseases under the broad category of familial adenomatous polyposis (FAP). FAP is characterized by adenomatous polyps of the colon and rectum, but also of upper gastrointestinal tract (ampullary, duodenal and gastric adenomas). FAP is a viciously premalignant disease with one or more polyps progressing through dysplasia to malignancy in untreated gene carriers with a median age at diagnosis of 40 years. Disease-associated mutations tend to be

clustered in the mutation cluster region (see below) and result in a truncated protein product.
- FAP encompasses other disease syndromes with extra-colonic manifestations: Gardner Syndrome and Turcot Syndrome. In Gardner Syndrome, patients with mutated APC may develop the following extra-intestinal manifestations: cancers of stomach, duodenum, pancreas, biliary tree, and gallbladder; hepatoblastoma; desmoid tumors; osteomas and dental abnormalities; epidermoid cysts and other skin abnormalities. Turcot syndrome is an autosomal dominant disorder in which APC mutations lead to malignant tumors of the brain associated with multiple colorectal adenomas. Skin features include sebaceous cysts, hyperpigmented and cafe au lait spots.
- Defects in APC are also a cause of hereditary desmoid disease (HDD), an autosomal dominant disorder with 100% penetrance and possible variable expression among affected relatives. In HDD patients, multifocal fibromatosis of the paraspinal muscles, breast, occiput, arms, lower ribs, abdominal wall, and mesentery is observed.
- Somatic mutations: APC is one of the most frequently mutated genes in cancer. Alterations have been observed in tumors of small and large intestine, stomach, pancreas, liver, soft tissues, urinary tract, ovary, adrenal gland, thyroid, upper aerodigestive tract... Over 60% of somatic mutations occur within the "mutation cluster region" (amino acids 1286-1513), with a very high frequency of alteration at amino acid 1450.

Both copies of the APC gene are mutated in 80% of sporadic colorectal tumors. Sporadic colorectal cancer is the third most frequent cancer in the world. Loss of normal APC function is known to be an early event in both familial and sporadic colorectal cancer, occurring at the pre-adenoma stage.

ATM (11q22-q23)
Ataxia Telangiectasia Mutated

Function
ATM (Derheimer and Kastan 2010) encodes a serine/threonine protein kinase that is recruited and activated by DNA double-strand breaks. It phosphorylates several key proteins that initiate activation of the DNA damage checkpoint, leading to cell cycle arrest, DNA repair or apoptosis.

Several of these targets, including p53, Chek2 and H2AX are tumor suppressors.

Cancer-Related Gene Alterations
- Various types of ATM germline mutations have been described, dispersed throughout the gene, and therefore most patients are compound heterozygotes; most mutations appear to inactivate the ATM protein by truncation, large deletions, or annulation of initiation or termination, although missense mutations have been described in the "PI3 kinase domain" and the "leucine zipper motif". Missense mutations outside these domains have been described among breast cancer patients.

- Defects in ATM are the cause of ataxia telangiectasia (AT). This rare recessive disorder is characterized by progressive cerebellar ataxia, dilation of the blood vessels in the conjunctiva and eyeballs, immunodeficiency, growth retardation and sexual immaturity.

  AT patients have a strong predisposition to cancer; about 30% of patients develop tumors, particularly lymphomas and leukemias. AT patients have an increased risk for breast cancer that has been ascribed to ATM's interaction and phosphorylation of BRCA1 and its associated proteins following DNA damage.

  Cells from affected individuals are highly sensitive to damage by ionizing radiations and resistant to inhibition of DNA synthesis following irradiation.

  The phenotypic manifestation of AT is due to the broad range of substrates for the ATM kinase, involving DNA repair, apoptosis, G1/S, intra-S checkpoint and G2/M checkpoints, gene regulation, translation initiation, and telomere maintenance. Therefore a defect in ATM has severe consequences in repairing certain types of damage to DNA, and cancer may result from improper repair.

- Somatic mutations have been observed in cancers of hematopoietic and lymphoid tissue (T-ALL, T-cell prolymphocytic leukemia, B-cell NHL, B-cell chronic lymphocytic leukemia (CLL)), ovary, lung, large intestine, stomach and upper aerodigestive tract.

  Biallelic mutation can occur in T-prolymphocytic leukemia. Most mutations are substitutions. No mutation hotspot has been described.

BAP1 (3p21.31-p21.2)
BRCA1 Associated Protein-1 (Ubiquitin Carboxy-Terminal Hydrolase)

Function
BAP1 encodes a deubiquitinating enzyme that plays a key role in chromatin structure. BAP1 acts as a tumor suppressor.

Cancer-Related Gene Alterations
- Germline BAP1 mutations have been associated with a novel cancer syndrome, characterized by malignant mesothelioma, uveal melanoma, cutaneous melanoma, and, possibly, by other cancers (Carbone et al. 2012)].
- Somatic mutations in BAP1 (mainly substitutions and deletions) are distributed throughout the gene and are notably observed in tumors affecting eye and pleura. A study found that BAP1 protein was inactivated in 15% of clear cell renal cell carcinoma (ccRCC).

  Mutations in BAP1 and PBRM1 were anticorrelated in ccRCC, and combined loss of BAP1 and PBRM1 in a few RCCs was associated with rhabdoid features. BAP1 loss was associated with high tumor grade (Peña-Llopis et al. 2012).

BLM (15q26.1)
Bloom Syndrome, RecQ Helicase-Like

Function

BLM (Chu and Hickson 2009) encodes a protein that has both DNA-stimulated ATPase and ATP-dependent DNA 3'-5' helicase activities. It may act to suppress inappropriate DNA recombination. Mutations causing Bloom syndrome disable the helicase activity.

BLM participates in a supercomplex of BRCA1-associated proteins named BASC (BRCA1-Associated genome Surveillance Complex) containing ATM (defective in ataxia telangiectasia), NBS1 (defective in Nijmegen syndrome) and MRE11 (defective in ataxia telangiectasia-like disorder), MLH1, MSH2 and MSH6 (which are involved in human non-polyposis colorectal cancer), RAD50 and DNA replication factor C.

Cancer-Related Gene Alterations
- Defects in BLM are the cause of Bloom syndrome (BS). BS is an autosomal recessive disorder characterized by proportionate pre- and postnatal growth deficiency, sun-sensitive telangiectatic hypo- and hyperpigmented skin and chromosomal instability. BS patients also show a very high incidence of cancers of most types (although lung and prostate cancers are rare), with a very early average age of onset (mean of 24 years of age). Leukemia predominates in childhood, and lymphomas and carcinomas appear during adolescence and early adulthood. Some normally rare tumors, such as osteosarcoma, Wilms tumor, medulloblastoma and meningioma, occur with a high prevalence in BS cases. The incidence of multiple neoplasms is also unusually high.
- A few BLM germline mutations have been described to date. They introduce either amino acid substitutions or premature nonsense codons into the coding sequence; one BLM mutation consisting in a 6 bp deletion accompanied by a 7 bp insertion at nucleic acid position 2281 is common in patients from Ashkenazi Jewish ancestry, leading to a truncated protein of 739 amino acids in length; two BLM mutations, 631delCAA and 1610insA were detected in Japanese patients.
- Somatic mutations are mainly substitutions. They are observed in tumors of large intestine. No mutation hotspot has been described.

BMPR1A (10q22.3)
Bone Morphogenetic Protein Receptor, Type IA

Function

BMPR1A encodes bone morphogenetic protein (BMP) receptor 1A, a serine/threonine kinase; its ligands are members of the TGF-β superfamily.

Cancer-Related Gene Alterations
- Mutations in BMPR1A (Bellam and Pasche 2010) are a cause of juvenile polyposis syndrome (JPS); also known as juvenile intestinal polyposis (JIP). JPS is an autosomal dominant gastrointestinal hamartomatous polyposis syndrome in which patients are at risk for developing gastrointestinal cancers. The lesions are typified by

a smooth histological appearance, predominant stroma, cystic spaces and lack of a smooth muscle core.
- Genetic defects in BMPR1A are a cause of Cowden disease (CD), an autosomal dominant cancer syndrome characterized by multiple hamartomas and by a high risk for breast, thyroid and endometrial cancers.
- Defects in BMPR1A are the cause of hereditary mixed polyposis syndrome 2 (HMPS2). Hereditary mixed polyposis syndrome (HMPS) is characterized by atypical juvenile polyps, colonic adenomas, and colorectal carcinomas.
- A microdeletion of chromosome 10q23 involving BMPR1A and PTEN is a cause of chromosome 10q23 deletion syndrome. The 10q23 microdeletion is also found in patients manifesting juvenile polyposis of infancy without cognitive disability.
- Somatic mutations observed in BMPR1A are substitutions only. Most of them are located in the protein kinase domain. They are rare, occurring in a small minority of stomach, kidney and large intestine tumors.

BRAF (7q34)
v-raf Murine Sarcoma Viral Oncogene Homolog B1

Function
BRAF (Röring and Brummer 2012) encodes a serine/threonine protein kinase (b-raf). Raf kinases are part of the Ras-MAPK signaling cascade. They phosphorylate MEK, which affects cell division, differentiation, and secretion.

Cancer-Related Gene Alterations
- No germinal BRAF mutations have been described to date.
- Somatic BRAF mutations have been found in various types of tumors, predominantly in malignant melanoma, colorectal tumors, low-grade ovarian serous carcinoma and thyroid papillary cancer; 80% of these mutations correspond to the hotspot transversion mutation T1799A that causes the amino acid substitution V600E. The other 20% accounts for a wide variable range of missense substitutions and all of them reside in the glycines of the G-loop in the exon 11 or in the activation segment in exon 15 near the V600. The mutation V600E confers transforming activity to the cells because it mimics the phosphorylation of T599 and/or S602 in the activation segment and so BRAF rests constitutively active in a Ras independent manner.
- V600E in BRAF is the most frequent oncogenic protein kinase mutation known.
- BRAF is mutated in 70% of malignant melanomas. The mutation V600E is an early event and alone is insufficient for the development of melanoma as it is present in 80% of primary melanomas and 80% of nevi, which are the first lesions associated with this tumor. No BRAF mutations are associated with uveal melanoma. In melanomas without BRAF mutation, alteration of NRAS (Q61R or Q61K) is often seen.
- In colorectal cancers, BRAF mutation V600E is associated with mismatch repair deficiency (MSI) and found in 40% of the cases while in mismatch repair proficient tumors (MSS) the frequency is around 5%. Gastric and endometrial MSI and MSS tumors do not have BRAF mutations. In tumors from the hereditary nonpolyposis

colorectal cancer (HNPCC), either with MLH1, MSH2 or MSH6 germline mutations or none, no BRAF mutations are detected. In colorectal tumors without BRAF mutation, an alteration of KRAS (G12C, G12D, G12V or G13D) is often seen.
- In ovarian and thyroid cancers, the only BRAF mutation present is V600E with a frequency around 30% and 50%, respectively.
- BRAF is involved in rare fusion events with AGTRAP (gastric cancer), AKAP9 (inv(7)(q21-22;q34) in papillary thyroid adenocarcinoma), FCHSD1 (t(5;7)(q31;q34) in congenital melanocytic nevus), SLC45A3 (prostate cancer), KIAA1549 (astrocytoma).

BRCA1 (17q21.31)
Breast Cancer 1, Early Onset

Function

BRCA1 (Roy et al. 2011) encodes a nuclear phosphoprotein that plays a role in maintaining genomic stability, and it also acts as a tumor suppressor. The encoded protein combines with other tumor suppressors, DNA damage sensors, and signal transducers to form a large multi-subunit protein complex known as the BRCA1-associated genome surveillance complex (BASC). BRCA1 associates with RNA polymerase II, and through the C-terminal domain, also interacts with histone deacetylase complexes. This protein thus plays a role in transcription, DNA repair of double-stranded breaks, and recombination.

BRCA1 has been implicated in two pathways of DNA double strand break repair: homologous recombination (HR) and non homologous end joining (NHEJ). Upon exposure to DNA damaging agents, BRCA1 becomes hyperphosphorylated and is rapidly relocated, along with Rad51, to sites of DNA synthesis marked by proliferating cell nuclear antigen (PCNA). Rad51 is a central player in HR, catalyzing the invasion of the single stranded DNA in a homologous duplex and facilitating the homology search during the establishment of joint molecules. Recent studies, however, have indicated that BRCA1 deficient breast cancer cells compensate for this deficiency by upregulating Rad51. The resultant HR may be erroneous and thereby lead to tumorigenesis. In addition, BRCA1 is said to inhibit the MRN complex which is implicated in bringing together two DNA strands together for the error prone NHEJ. BRCA1-deficient cells are sensitive to ionizing radiation and DNA damaging drugs, such as mitomycin C.

BRCA1 is required for FANCD2 targeting to sites of DNA damage (see Fanconi anemia pathway)

Cancer-Related Gene Alterations

- Defects in BRCA1 are a cause of susceptibility to breast-ovarian cancer familial type 1 (BROVCA1), a condition associated with familial predisposition to cancer of the breast and ovaries (for BROVCA2, see BRCA2; for BROVCA3, see RAD51C). Characteristic features in affected families are an early age of onset of breast cancer (often before age 50), increased chance of bilateral cancers (in both breasts/both ovaries, independently), frequent occurrence of breast cancer among men, increased incidence of tumors of other specific organs, such as colon and prostate. BRCA1 carries as many as 1,000 different disease associated mutations, many of which are rare. These mutations are distributed uniformly along the entire coding region and intronic sequences flanking each exon. Mutations at more than one locus can be involved in different families or even in the same case. Mutations in BRCA1 are at a high penetrance and are thought to be responsible for more than 80% of inherited breast-ovarian cancer and for 40% of inherited breast cancers.

- Defects in BRCA1 are a cause of susceptibility to ovarian cancer. The lifetime risks of ovarian cancer associated with a BRCA1 gene mutation carrier has been estimated as 40 to 50%.
- Somatic point mutations (deletions, insertions, substitutions, others) have been observed mostly in breast (2%) and ovarian (2%) tumors. There are no mutation hotspots.
- An increased relative risk to the development of cancer of the colon, cervix, uterus, pancreas and prostate has been suggested in BRCA1-mutation carriers.

BRCA2 (13q12-q13)
Breast Cancer 2, Early Onset

Function

BRCA2 (Roy et al. 2011)] is implicated in maintenance of genomic integrity and in cellular response to DNA damage. The BRCA2 protein interacts with the Rad51 recombinase to regulate homologous recombination (HR). CHEK1 and CHEK2 both phosphorylate the Rad51/BRCA2 complex and regulate the functional association of this complex in response to DNA damage.

BRCA2 is also implicated in cell cycle checkpoints. Following exposure to X-rays or UV light, cells expressing truncated BRCA2 protein are stopped in the G1 and G2/M phases.

Cancer-Related Gene Alterations

- Defects in BRCA2 are a cause of susceptibility to breast-ovarian cancer familial type 2 (BROVCA2), a condition associated with familial predisposition to cancer of the breast and ovaries (for BROVCA1, see BRCA1; for BROVCA3, see RAD51C). Mutations at more than one locus can be involved in different families or even in the same case. Characteristic features in affected families are an early age of onset of breast cancer (often before age 50), increased chance of bilateral cancers (cancer that develop in both breasts, or both ovaries, independently), frequent occurrence of breast cancer among men, increased incidence of tumors of other specific organs, such as the prostate, stomach, pharynx, gallbladder, bile duct, colon and pancreas. Cumulative risk of breast cancer in BRCA2 mutation carriers was estimated to 45% by the age of 70 years while ovarian cancer risk in carriers was estimated to 11%.
- Somatic mutations in BRCA2 (substitutions, insertions, deletions) are infrequent in sporadic breast cancer. Loss of heterozygosity at the BRCA2 locus has been frequently found in sporadic breast and ovarian tumors.
- Biallelic mutations of the BRCA2 gene are the cause of Fanconi anemia complementation group D type 1 (FANCD1) (see Fanconi anemia pathway). Fanconi anemia (FA) is an autosomal recessive disorder affecting all bone marrow elements and associated with cardiac, renal and limb malformations as well as dermal

pigmentary changes. The FANCD1 and FANCN (see Fanconi anemia pathway and PALB2) subgroups are clinically different from other FA subgroups as these subgroups are associated with increased predisposition to solid childhood malignancies such as medulloblastoma and Wilms tumor.

At the cellular level, FA is a chromosomal fragility syndrome. FA cells are hypersensitive to DNA interstrand crosslinking agents and also show an increased number of spontaneous breaks.

Note: information regarding breast cancer and BRCA2 mutations and polymorphisms are available in a central repository formed by the National Human Genome Research; National Institute of Health. This repository, named Breast Cancer Information Core (BIC) - NHGRI, is available at the following address: http://research.nhgri.nih.gov/bic/

BRIP1 (17q23.2)
BRCA1 Interacting Protein C-Terminal Helicase 1 (BRIP1) or Fanconi Anemia, Complementation Group J (FANCJ)

Function
The protein encoded by BRIP1 (Cantor and Guillemette 2011) is a DNA-dependent ATPase and a 5' to 3' DNA helicase required for the maintenance of chromosomal stability. This protein acts late in the Fanconi anemia pathway, after FANCD2 ubiquitination (see Fanconi anemia pathway). It is involved in the repair of DNA double-strand breaks by homologous recombination in a manner that depends on its association with BRCA1.

Cancer-Related Gene Alterations
- Defects in BRIP1 are a cause of low-risk susceptibility to breast cancer.
- Defects in BRIP1 are the cause of Fanconi anemia complementation group J (FANCJ) (see Fanconi anemia pathway)

BUB1B (15q15)
Budding Uninhibited By Benzimidazoles 1 Homolog Beta

Function
BUB1B (Wan et al. 2012) encodes a kinase involved in spindle checkpoint function. The protein has been localized to the kinetochore and plays a role in the inhibition of the anaphase-promoting complex/cyclosome, delaying the onset of anaphase and ensuring proper chromosome segregation. Impaired spindle checkpoint function has been found in many forms of cancer.

Cancer-Related Gene Alterations
- Defects in BUB1B are the cause of mosaic variegated aneuploidy syndrome (MVA). MVA is a severe autosomal recessive developmental disorder characterized by mosaic aneuploidies, predominantly trisomies and monosomies, involving multiple

different chromosomes and tissues. The proportion of aneuploid cells varies but is usually more than 25% and is substantially greater than in normal individuals. Affected individuals typically present with severe intrauterine growth retardation and microcephaly. Eye anomalies, mild dysmorphism, variable developmental delay, and a broad spectrum of additional congenital abnormalities and medical conditions may also occur. The risk of malignancy is high, with rhabdomyosarcoma, Wilms tumor and leukemia reported in several cases. MVA is caused by biallelic mutations in the BUB1B gene. Each family carries one missense mutation and one mutation that results in premature protein truncation or an absent transcript.

CASP8 (2q33-q34)
Caspase 8, Apoptosis-Related Cysteine Peptidase

Function
CASP8 (Fulda 2009) encodes caspase 8, a member of the cysteine-aspartic acid protease (caspase) family. Sequential activation of caspases plays a central role in the execution-phase of cell apoptosis. Initiator caspases, such as caspase 8, may be directly activated by death receptors such as FasR.

Cancer-Related Gene Alterations
- Somatic mutations (mostly missense and nonsense substitutions) in CASP8 are found in colon and upper aerodigestive tract tumors. They are also observed in a small percentage of breast tumors.

CBFB (16q22.1)
Core-Binding Factor, Beta Subunit

Function
Protein CBF is a heterodimer comprising the subunit b (CBFb, encoded by CBFB) and the subunit CBFa. CBFa binds to a core motif of the DNA; CBFb increases CBFa's affinity to DNA by 5 to 10 fold; CBF is a transcription factor which regulates the expression of myeloid and T-cell specific genes such as: GM-CSF, M-CSFR, IL3, T- Cell receptors TCRA-D, TCRB and TCRG; CBF cooperate with various tissue specific factors to activate these lineage-restricted transcriptions; homozygous knock down of either CBFb or CBFa results in embryonic lethality, showing that they are essential for fetal liver hematopoiesis

Cancer-Related Gene Alterations
- Chromosomal aberrations: inv(16)(p13q22), t(16;16)(p13;q22), and del(16)(q22) are associated with acute myeloid leukemia (AML) or myelodysplastic syndromes (MDS). The hybrid gene generated is CBFB-MYH11, in which the N-terminus and most of CBFB is fused to the MYH11 C-terminus (Tirado et al. 2010).

CBL (11q23.3)
Cas-Br-M (Murine) Ecotropic Retroviral Transforming Sequence

Function

CBL encodes a protein with negative regulatory activity in protein tyrosine kinase-mediated signaling pathways; CBL may inhibit cell growth resulting from activation of the EGF, PDGF and CSF1 receptors by marking these receptors for ubiquitination and subsequent degradation.

Cancer-Related Gene Alterations
- Germinal alterations: the fragile site FRA11B has been localized to a stretch of CCG trinucleotides found in the 5' part of the CBL gene and has been involved in the pathogenesis of a proportion of inherited Jacobsen syndromes which have a del(11)(q23qter) telomeric of an expansion of the stretch of CCG triplets
- Sporadic alterations: an extension of an ATG trinucleotide repeat with no translation shift was detected in the coding region of CBL in 9% of the genetically unstable sporadic gastrointestinal tumors,
- Somatic CBL mutations have been found in some hematopoietic/lymphoid tissue and lung cancers. Most mutations are substitution missense and are related to a protein region located between amino acids 360 and 460 (Ogawa et al. 2010).

CDH1 (16q22.1)
Cadherin 1, Type 1, E-Cadherin (Epithelial)

Function

One of the most important and ubiquitous types of adhesive interactions required for the maintenance of solid tissues is that mediated by the classic cadherin adhesion molecules. Cadherins are transmembrane Ca2+- dependent homophilic adhesion receptors that are well known to play important roles in cell recognition and cell sorting during development. However, they continue to be expressed at high levels in virtually all solid tissues. There are many members of the classic cadherin family (which is a subset of the larger cadherin superfamily), but E-cadherin (encoded by CDH1) in epithelial tissues has been the most studied in the context of stable adhesions. Continued expression and functional activity of E-cadherin are required for cells to remain tightly associated in the epithelium, and in its absence the many other cell adhesion and cell junction proteins expressed in epithelial cells are not capable of supporting intercellular adhesion. In its capacity to maintain the overall state of adhesion between epithelial cells, E-cadherin is thought to act as an important suppressor of epithelial tumor cell invasiveness and metastasis.

Cancer-Related Gene Alterations
- Defects in CDH1 are a cause of hereditary familial diffuse gastric cancer (HDGC). Dozens of CDH1 germline mutations have been described in HDGC families (Moran et al. 2005).
  Most are inactivating (frameshift, nonsense, and splice-site); the remainders are missense. The mutations are distributed equally throughout the gene.

- Defects in CDH1 are found in gastric, breast, biliary tract, colorectal, thyroid and ovarian cancers.

  Frequent somatic mutations (50%) in CDH have been identified in sporadic diffuse gastric cancer (DGC). Most mutations are missense (exons 8, 9) or exon skipping. In most cases, CDH1 mutations are found in combination with loss of the wild-type allele. Somatic mutations in CDH1 are found in about 56% of lobular breast tumors, generally (>90%) in combination with loss of the wild-type allele, while no mutations were found in ductal primary breast carcinomas. Most of these somatic mutations result in premature stop codons as a consequence of insertions, deletions and nonsense mutations leading to the loss of the CDH1 cell-cell adhesion functionality.

  Other cancer-confined E-cadherin mutations also result in crippled proteins. The distinctive invasive growth pattern, which is typical for lobular breast cancers, is fully compatible with this functional inactivation.

CDK4 (11q23.3)
Cyclin-Dependent Kinase 4

Function

CDK4 encodes the catalytic subunit of a heterodimeric serine/threonine protein kinase which is involved in controlling progression through the G1 phase of the cell cycle. The activating partner of CDK4 (the regulatory subunit) is one of the D-type cyclins: CCND1, CCND2 or CCND3.

Once activated, the CDK4-cyclin D complex phosphorylates members of the retinoblastoma protein family (pRb, p107, p130).

The activity of CDK4 is inhibited by the p16/INK4A (encoded by CDKN2A) protein, which interferes with the cyclin D-binding region.

Cancer-Related Gene Alterations

- Germline mutations in the CDK4 gene have so far only been found in families with inherited malignant melanoma (familial cutaneous malignant melanoma 3 or CMM3) and multiple atypical nevi. There are six such families reported. The mutations affect the arginine encoded by codon 24, changing it either to cysteine (two families) or to histidine (four families).
- Somatic alterations: amplification of the chromosomal region that includes CDK4 and CDK4 overexpression is commonly seen in gliomas and several subgroups of sarcomas (in particular liposarcoma, alveolar rhabdomyosarcoma and osteosarcoma), and may also occur in other tumors such as malignant melanoma (cases with wild-type BRAF and NRAS genes), and carcinomas of the breast, colon, lung, ovary and oral cavity. Point mutations have only rarely been observed and are of unknown biological significance.

CDKN1B (12p13.1-p12)
Cyclin-Dependent Kinase Inhibitor 1B (P27, Kip1)

Function

CDKN1B (Lee and Kim 2009) encodes a cyclin-dependent kinase inhibitor, which shares a limited similarity with CDK inhibitor CDKN1A/p21. The protein binds to and prevents the activation of cyclin E-CDK2 or cyclin D-CDK4 complexes, and thus controls the cell cycle progression at G1. The degradation of this protein, which is triggered by its CDK dependent phosphorylation and subsequent ubiquitination by Skp, Cullin, F-box (SCF) complexes, is required for the cellular transition from quiescence to the proliferative state.

Cancer-Related Gene Alterations

- Compared to CDKN2A, CDKN1B is less frequently altered in tumors. Somatic mutations (missense substitutions or deletions) have been observed in breast and ovarian tumors.

CDKN2A (9p21)
Cyclin-Dependent Kinase Inhibitor 2A (Melanoma, P16, Inhibits CDK4)

Function

CDKN2A (Kim and Sharpless 2006) encodes p16-INK4a, a protein that interacts strongly with cyclin-dependent kinases (CDK)4 and CDK6 and inhibits their ability to interact with cyclins D. P16-INK4a is capable of inducing cell cycle arrest in G1 and G2 phases. It acts as a tumor suppressor.

Cancer-Related Gene Alterations

- CDKN2A is one of the most frequently altered genes in tumors. Somatic deletions and/or mutations of various types have been observed in tumors of the following tissues (among others): genital tract, pleura, pancreas, biliary tract, skin, upper aerodigestive tract, CNS, esophagus, urinary tract... Somatic mutations have been found throughout the gene.
- Among skin tumors, CDKN2A alterations are highly associated with cutaneous melanoma (while they are rare in uveal melanoma) and several melanoma-associated syndromes, such as:
  - Cutaneous malignant melanoma type 2 (CMM2). This syndrome arises *de novo* or from a pre-existing benign nevus, which occurs most often in the skin but also may involve other sites. CMM2 is transmitted as an autosomal dominant trait;
  - Familial atypical multiple mole melanoma carcinoma syndrome (FAMMM), in which patients have an increased risk of developing melanoma and other malignant neoplasms, for example, a pancreatic cancer (FAMMMPC). Germline CDKN2A mutations are found in approximately 40% of the FAMMM syndrome patients;
  - Melanoma-astrocytoma syndrome, which is characterized by a dual predisposition to melanoma and neural system tumors, commonly astrocytoma.

- Genetic defects in CDKN2A may also be a cause of Li-Fraumeni syndrome (LFS). LFS is a highly penetrant familial cancer phenotype usually associated with inherited mutations in TP53.

CEBPA (19q13.1)
CCAAT/Enhancer Binding Protein (C/EBP), Alpha (A)

Function
C/EBPα, the protein encoded by CEBPA (Paz-Priel and Friedman 2011)], plays important roles in lineage determination and gene activation in a variety of cell types by activating transcription from lineage-specific promoters. In hematopoiesis, C/EBPα drives granulocytic differentiation of myelocytic cells. C/EBPα is also a key factor for hepatocyte and adipocyte development. A truncated form (30 kDa) is frequently observed. Both isoforms can be detected within the cell and it is likely that the ratio of isoforms is important in mediating proliferation and differentiation control.

Cancer-Related Gene Alterations
- Germline mutations in CEBPA have been described in 2 familial cases of AML.
- A number of different somatic mutations in CEBPA have been detected in cancer. They tend to cluster to two regions. The first group affects the N-terminal region of C/EBPα. These mutations are often insertions or deletions which cause frameshifts leading to premature truncation of the protein. In this case, translation is reinitiated at an internal ATG and the 30kDa protein, which lacks the first transactivating domain, is produced.
Secondly, in-frame or missense mutations occur within the C-terminal region of C/EBPα, disrupting the basic zipper region and thus affecting DNA binding, protein interactions as well as homo and heterodimerization with other C/EBP family members.
- Mutations in CEBPA occur in approximately 10% of all AML and are associated with normal karyotype AML. These mutations tend to confer favorable prognosis. The involvement of CEBPA mutations in familial cases of AML, along with evidence of mutations persisting between presentation and relapse indicate that mutations in CEBPA are an early event in leukemogenesis.
- In rare cases, CEBPA has been found to be mutated in MDS, lung tumors and prostate tumors.
- A t(14;19)(q32;q13) translocation leading to the IGH@-CEBPA fusion has been rarely observed in B-cell precursor acute lymphoblastic leukemia (BCP-ALL)

CHEK2 (22q12.1)
CHK2 Checkpoint Homolog (S. Pombe)

Function
CHEK2-encoded protein, Chk2 (Antoni et al. 2007), regulates cell cycle checkpoints and apoptosis, especially in response to DNA double-strand breaks. Activated Chk2 may

phosphorylate various targets, among which p53, Cdc25a, PML and Brca1, ultimately leading to cell cycle arrest and DNA repair.

Cancer-Related Gene Alterations
- Germline mutations: the northern European founder mutation "1100delC" is the most common found in breast cancer families. Other small deletions, stops, and missense mutations, such as Arg145Trp and Ile157Thr are rare in cancer families but not found in controls.
  The 1100delC mutation appears to increase the penetrance of mutations in certain other breast cancer genes, notably BRCA2.
- Somatic mutations: missense mutations in the CHEK2 FHA and kinase domains as well as frameshifts and nonsense mutations have been found at low frequencies in osteosarcoma and more rarely in carcinomas of the ovary, lung, and vulva.

CTNNB1 (3p21)
Catenin (Cadherin-Associated Protein), Beta 1, 88kda

Function

Beta (β)-catenin, the protein encoded by CTNNB1 (Clevers and Nusse 2012) has important functions in the E-cadherin-mediated cell-cell adhesion system and also as a downstream signaling molecule in the Wnt pathway.

Cytoplasmic accumulation of β-catenin allows it to translocate to the nucleus to form complexes with transcription factors of the T cell factor-lymphoid enhancer factor (Tcf-Lef) family. β-catenin is assumed to transactivate mostly unknown target genes, which may stimulate cell proliferation or inhibit apoptosis.

The β-catenin level in the cell is regulated by its association with the adenomatous polyposis coli (APC) tumor suppressor protein, axin and GSK-3b.

Phosphorylation of β-catenin by the APC-axin-GSK-3b complex leads to its degradation by the ubiquitin-proteasome system.

Cancer-Related Gene Alterations
- Somatic point mutations have been observed in various (almost all) types of cancers, with high levels (>20%) in cancers of soft tissues, pancreas, pituitary, liver, endometrium, adrenal glands, colon. β-catenin alterations may facilitate the development of hepatocellular carcinoma in the course of chronic hepatitis. Somatic mutations are observed mostly in regions corresponding to the first 75 amino acids. Substitution hotspots (missense, in most cases) correspond to amino acids 34, 37, 40, 45.
- Of note, a chromosomal aberration involving CTNNB1 is found in salivary gland pleiomorphic adenomas, the most common benign epithelial tumors of the salivary gland. Translocation t(3;8)(p21;q12) fuses a portion of CTNNB1 with PLAG1.

CYLD (16q12.1)
Cylindromatosis (Turban Tumor Syndrome)

Function

CYLD (Massoumi 2011) encodes a cytoplasmic protein that functions as a deubiquitinating enzyme. It is a negative regulator of various signaling pathways, including TRAF2 and NFκB signaling pathways.

Cancer-related gene alterations
- Mutations in CYLD have been associated with familial cylindromatosis, multiple familial trichoepithelioma, and Brooke-Spiegler syndrome:
  - Familial cylindromatosis is an autosomal dominant and highly tumor type-specific disorder. The tumors (known as cylindromas because of their characteristic microscopic architecture) are believed to arise from or recapitulate the appearance of the eccrine or apocrine cells of the skin that secrete sweat and scent respectively. Cylindromas arise predominantly in hairy parts of the body with approximately 90% on the head and neck. The development of a confluent mass which may ulcerate or become infected has led to the designation 'turban tumor syndrome'. The skin tumors show differentiation in the direction of hair structures, hence the synonym trichoepithelioma.
  - Multiple familial trichoepithelioma is an autosomal dominant dermatosis characterized by the presence of many skin tumors predominantly on the face. Since histologic examination shows dermal aggregates of basaloid cells with connection to or differentiation toward hair follicles, this disorder has been thought to represent a benign hamartoma of the pilosebaceous apparatus. Trichoepitheliomas can degenerate into basal cell carcinoma.
  - Brooke-Spiegler syndrome is an autosomal dominant disorder characterized by the appearance of multiple skin appendage tumors such as cylindroma, trichoepithelioma, and spiradenoma. These tumors are typically located in the head and neck region, appear in early adulthood, and gradually increase in size and number throughout life.
- Among tumors, somatic CYLD alterations, mostly substitutions or insertions, have been observed only in skin tumors. No specific mutation hotspot has been described to date.

DNMT3A (2p23)
DNA (Cytosine-5-)-Methyltransferase 3 Alpha

Function

DNA methyltransferase (DNMT) add methyl groups to DNA to effect gene expression (Chédin 2011). There are three types of DNMTs. DNMT1 is predominately responsible for hemimethylated CpG island methylation, DNMT2 in fact transfers methyl groups to RNA not DNA, hence has been renamed to tRNA aspartic acid methyltransferase 1 (TRDMT1) and DNMT3 is responsible for unmethylated CpG island methylation. The DNMT3 family comprises the two active DNMT3A and DNMT3B enzymes.

Cancer-Related Gene Alterations
- Somatic mutations in DNMT3A have been observed mainly in tumors of hematopoietic and lymphoid tissue and of large intestine. They are missense substitutions (80%), with a mutation hotspot at amino acid 882.

EGFR (7p12)
Epidermal Growth Factor Receptor

Function

Epidermal growth factor receptor (Seshacharyulu 2012), the protein encoded by EGFR exists on the cell surface and is activated by binding of its specific ligands, including epidermal growth factor (EGF) and transforming growth factor α (TGFα). Upon activation by its growth factor ligands, EGFR undergoes a transition from an inactive monomeric form to an active homodimer. In addition to forming homodimers after ligand binding, EGFR may pair with another member of the ErbB receptor family, such as ErbB2/Her2/neu, to create an activated heterodimer. EGFR downstream signaling proteins initiate several signal transduction cascades, principally the MAPK, Akt and JNK pathways, thus modulating phenotypes such as cell migration, adhesion, and proliferation.

Cancer-Related Gene Alterations
- Somatic EGFR mutations have been associated mainly with lung cancer. They have also been observed in a small minority (<7%) of other tumors, such as those of adrenal glands, CNS, prostate, thyroid…Mutations are mostly substitutions (about 50%) and deletions (about 33%). Many mutation events occur in a region corresponding to amino acids 700-870. There is a substitution hotspot at amino acid 858. Complex mutation events have a hotspot at amino acids 746-750.

ERBB2 (17q11.2-q12)
v-erb-b2 Erythroblastic Leukemia Viral Oncogene Homolog 2, Neuro/Glioblastoma Derived Oncogene Homolog (Avian)

Function

ERBB2 encodes a member of the epidermal growth factor receptor (EGFR) family of receptor tyrosine kinases. This protein has no ligand binding domain of its own and therefore cannot bind growth factors. However, it does bind tightly to other ligand-bound EGF receptor family members to form a heterodimer, stabilizing ligand binding and enhancing kinase-mediated activation of downstream signaling pathways, such as those involving mitogen-activated protein kinase and phosphatidylinositol-3 kinase.

Cancer-Related Gene Alterations
- ERBB2 is commonly amplified in primary breast cancer (25%-30% of cases), defining a specific class of tumors frequently treated with compounds trastuzumab, pertuzumab and lapatinib.

- ERBB2 is also amplified (and overexpressed) in bladder carcinomas, in Barrett carcinoma, ovarian cancer, carcinoma of the salivary glands, endometrial, gastric, and prostate cancers. ERBB2 overexpression (without gene amplification) is observed in tumors of various other types.
- Somatic point mutations (mainly substitutions and insertions) are observed in cancers of endometrium, stomach, CNS (glioblastoma), liver, ovary, breast, large intestine, lung and pancreas. These mutations impact the tyrosine kinase activity.

EXT1 (8q24.11) and EXT2 (11p11.2)
Echinoderm Microtubule Associated Protein Like 4

Function

The gene products of EXT1 and EXT2 are endoplasmic reticulum localized type II transmembrane glycoproteins. *In vivo*, they form a stable hetero-oligomeric complex that accumulates in the Golgi apparatus, where it is involved in heparan sulphate proteoglycan (HSPG) biosynthesis. The EXT1/EXT2 complex catalyses the elongation of the HS chain, which is subsequently deacetylated, sulphated and epimerized resulting in a large spectrum of structural heterogenic HS chains. The sulphation pattern of HS chains is critical for binding specific proteins. Several growth factors have conserved patterns of basic amino acids for binding to HSPGs, which is crucial for proper signaling.

Cancer-related gene alterations
- Germline alterations in EXT1 and EXT2 are a cause of hereditary multiple exostoses (HME) type 1 and type II, respectively (Wuyts and Van Hul 2000). HME is a heterogeneous autosomal dominant disorder primarily affecting endochondral bone during growth. The disease is characterized by formation of numerous cartilage-capped, benign bone tumors (osteocartilaginous exostoses or osteochondromas) that are often accompanied by skeletal deformities and short stature. In a small percentage of cases exostoses have exhibited malignant transformation resulting in an osteosarcoma or chondrosarcoma. Osteochondromas development can also occur as a sporadic event. EXT1 mutations include nucleotide substitutions (54%), small deletions (27%) and small insertions (16%), of which the majority is predicted to result in a truncated or non-functional protein. EXT2 mutations include nucleotide substitutions (57%), small deletions (19%) and small insertions (24%), of which the majority is predicted to result in a truncated or non-functional protein.
- Defects in EXT1 are the cause of multiple exostoses observed in Langer-Giedon syndrome (LGS; also known as trichorhinophalangeal syndrome type 2 (TRPS2). It is a contiguous gene syndrome due to deletions in chromosome 8q24.1 and resulting in the loss of functional copies of EXT1 and TRPS1.
- Defects in EXT1 are a cause of chondrosarcoma, ranging from slow-growing non-metastasizing lesions to highly aggressive metastasizing sarcomas.
- Defects in EXT2 are the cause of multiple exostoses observed in Potocki-Shaffer syndrome. It is a contiguous gene syndrome due to proximal deletion of chromosome 11p11.2, including EXT2 and ALX4 (ALX homeobox 4).

- No EXT1/EXT2 somatic mutations were found in 34 sporadic and hereditary osteochondromas and secondary peripheral chondrosarcomas tested.

Fanconi Anemia pathway

FANCA (16q24.3) and **FANCB** (Xp22.2) and **FANCC** (9q22.3) and **FANCD1 (BRCA2)** (13q12-q13) and **FANCD2** (3p25.3) and **FANCE** (6p21-22) and **FANCF** (11p15) and **FANCG** (9p13) and **FANCI** (15q26.1) and **FANCJ (BRIP1)** (17q23.2) and **FANCL** (2p16.1) and **FANCM** (14q21.2) and **PALB2 (FANCN)** (16p12.2) and **RAD51C (FANCO)** (17q25.1) and **BRCA1** (17q21.31)

Fanconi anemia, complementation group A and Fanconi anemia, complementation group B and Fanconi anemia, complementation group C and Fanconi anemia, complementation group D1/Breast cancer 2, early onset and Fanconi anemia, complementation group D2 and Fanconi anemia, complementation group E and Fanconi anemia, complementation group F and Fanconi anemia, complementation group G and Fanconi anemia, complementation group I and Fanconi anemia, complementation group J/ BRCA1 interacting protein C-terminal helicase 1 and Fanconi anemia, complementation group L and Fanconi anemia, complementation group M and Partner and localizer of BRCA2/Fanconi anemia, complementation group N and RAD51 homolog C (S. cerevisiae)/ Fanconi anemia, complementation group O and Breast cancer 1, early onset.

Function

The proteins encoded by these genes function in a common DNA repair signaling pathway, the Fanconi Anemia (FA) pathway, which closely cooperates with other DNA repair proteins for resolving DNA interstrand cross-links (ICLs) during DNA replication. ICLs are among the most deleterious DNA lesions, since they block DNA replication and transcription. DNA ICLs can be caused by endogenous sources such as nitrous acid and aldehydes, or exogenous agents such as cisplatin and its derivatives.

A central event in the resolution of DNA ICLs is the monoubiquitination of FANCD2 and FANCI upon DNA damage, which is mediated by a group of upstream FA proteins (FANCA, FANCB, FANCC, FANCE, FANCF, FANCG, FANCL, and FANCM) that are assembled into a large nuclear E3 ubiquitin ligase complex, termed the "FA core complex" (Kennedy and D'Andrea 2005; Wang 2007).

The monoubiquitinated FANCD2/FANCI heterodimer was shown to play multiple roles in the pathway (Knipscheer et al. 2009), and to functionally interact with downstream FA proteins such as FANCD1 (or BRCA2), FANCN (or PALB2), and FANCJ (or BRIP1), and their associated proteins, BRCA1 or RAD51C.

Cancer-Related Gene Alterations
- FA is caused by mutations in at least 13 distinct genes (FANCA, FANCB, FANCC, FANCD1, FANCD2, FANCE, FANCF, FANCG, FANCI, FANCJ, FANCL,

FANCM, and FANCN). About 66% of FA cases are caused by mutations in FANCA, 10% by mutations in FANCC and 10% by mutations in FANCG.
- In FA genes, various germinal alterations (nucleotide substitutions, deletions, or insertions) have been described. Somatic point mutations are rare.
- Principal cancers observed in biallelic mutation carriers (phenotype of FA patients) are acute myeloid leukemia, head and neck squamous cell carcinoma, anogenital tumors. In the case of biallelic mutation in FANCD1/BRCA2 or FANCN/PALB2, aggressive FA may be observed, associated to childhood solid tumors (Wilms tumor and medulloblastoma).
- In carriers of monoallelic mutation, only those with alteration in FANCD1/BRCA2 are highly susceptible to (breast) cancer, while carriers of FANCJ/BRIP1 or FANCN/PALB2 have a low-risk of developing breast cancer.

FAM123B (Xq11.2)
Family with Sequence Similarity 123B

Function
FAM123B (Kim et al. 2011) encodes a protein associating with β–catenin (see CTNNB1), axin1, β-transducin repeat-containing protein 2 (β-TrCP2) and APC (see APC) to negatively regulate the Wnt signaling pathway (by promoting the ubiquitination and degradation of β-catenin). It also plays a role in the recruitment of APC from microtubules to the plasma membrane and appears to be involved in the maintenance of intercellular junctions. FAM123B enhances transcription activation by the Wilms tumor protein (see WT1).

Cancer-related Gene Alterations
- Somatic tumor-specific FAM123B mutations have been observed in kidney and colorectal cancers and in acute myeloid leukemia. In Wilms tumors, the most commonly observed mutation is the deletion of the entire FAM123B gene. Truncation mutations and missense mutations have also been observed. 7-29% of Wilms tumors show deletions or mutations of FAM123B. Inactivating mutations in FAM123B (deletions and truncating/frameshift mutations) appear to be negatively correlated in Wilms tumors with activating mutations in exon 3 of CTNNB1 (encoding β-catenin), implicating the activation of the Wnt signaling pathway in the formation of Wilms tumors since both inactivating mutations of FAM123B and activating mutations of CTNNB1 function to activate this signaling pathway.

FBXW7 (4q31.3)
F-Box and WD Repeat Domain Containing 7

Function
FBXW7 (Welcker and Clurman 2008) encodes a member of the F-box protein family which is characterized by an approximately 40 amino acid motif, the F-box. The F-box proteins constitute one of the four subunits of ubiquitin protein ligase complex called SCFs

(SKP1-cullin-F-box), which function in phosphorylation-dependent ubiquitination. This protein binds directly to cyclin E and probably targets cyclin E for ubiquitin-mediated degradation.

Cancer-related Gene Alterations
- Somatic mutations, consisting mostly in substitutions, have been observed in tumors of biliary tract, endometrium, hematopoietic and lymphoid tissue, large intestine, thyroid, stomach and cervix. Mutations have also been described in ovarian and breast cancer cell lines. Mutations are present throughout the gene, but hotspots are found at amino acids 465, 479 and 505.

FGFR3 (4p16.3)
Fibroblast Growth Factor Receptor 3

Function
FGFR3 encodes a member of the fibroblast growth factor receptor (FGFR) family with tyrosine kinase activity; binding of ligand (fibroblast growth factor –FGF-) induces receptor dimerization, autophosphorylation and signal transduction.

FGFR family members differ from one another in their ligand affinities and tissue distribution.

This particular family member binds acidic and basic FGF and plays a role in bone development and maintenance.

Mutations in this gene lead to craniosynostosis and multiple types of skeletal dysplasia. Three alternatively spliced transcript variants that encode different protein isoforms have been described.

Cancer-Related Gene Alterations
- Somatic mutations in the FGFR3 gene are mainly associated with bladder cancer (Knowles 2007).
  These mutations overactivate the FGFR3 protein, which likely directs bladder cells to grow and divide abnormally. In addition to bladder cancer, somatic FGFR3 mutations have been associated with multiple myeloma (MM) and cervical cancer. In MM, a t(4;14)(p16.3;q32.3) translocation leading to a FGFR3-IgH fusion gene has been observed. Mutations that have been associated with cervical cancer are point mutations, mainly substitutions, in FGFR3.
- FGFR3 mutations that lead to multiple myeloma and cervical cancer are thought to overactivate the FGFR3 protein.
- The same FGFR3 mutations known from bladder carcinoma have been shown to cause benign human skin tumors such as seborrheic keratoses and epidermal nevi.
- Somatic mutation hotspots: substitutions at codons 249 (S249C), 373 (Y373C) and 248 (R248C)

FH (1q42.1)
Fumarate Hydratase (Fumarase)

Function

Fumarase (Yogev et al. 2010) is a homotetramer that plays a key enzymatic role in fundamental metabolic pathways. The mitochondrial isoenzyme catalyzes conversion of fumarate to malate in the Krebs, or tricarboxylic acid cycle, in which acetyl-CoA produces CO_2, reduced electron carriers ($FADH_2$ and NADH) and ATP. The cytosolic isoenzyme is involved with amino acid metabolism.

Cancer-related Gene Alterations
- Germline mutations in FH are associated with two distinct conditions:
  - Homozygous and compound heterozygous mutations (e.g., missense and in-frame deletions) of the 3' end result in fumarate hydratase deficiency (FHD). FHD is characterized by progressive encephalopathy, developmental delay, hypotonia, cerebral atrophy and lactic and pyruvic acidemia. The most common allelic abnormality is a 3 base pair- AAA insertion.
  - Heterozygous 5' mutations (e.g., nonsense, missense and deletions ranging from one base pair to whole gene) predispose individuals to somatic mutations in the normal allele leading to hereditary leiomyomatosis and renal cell carcinoma / multiple cutaneous and uterine leiomyomatosis (HLRCC/MCUL1).
- Somatic mutations: loss-of-heterozygosity of the wild type allele results in functional nullizygosity for fumarate hydratase. Malignant uterine and kidney tumors characteristic of HLRCC can subsequently develop. Uterine leiomyomatosis has also been observed in patients with deletion of FH from structural rearrangements of 1q42.1. The probable mechanism is presumably haploinsufficiency

FLCN (17p11.2)
Folliculin

Function

Folliculin forms a complex with folliculin-interacting proteins 1 and 2 (FNIP1 and FNIP2), and 5'-AMP-activated protein kinase (AMPK), an important energy sensor in cells that negatively regulates mammalian target of rapamycin (mTOR). Folliculin plays a role in the regulation of key molecules in TGF-β signaling. Folliculin is a tumor suppressor.

Cancer-Related Gene Alterations
- Defects in FLCN are the cause of Birt-Hogg-Dube syndrome (BHD) (Toro et al. 2008). BHD is a rare autosomal dominant genodermatosis characterized by hair follicle hamartomas (fibrofolliculomas), kidney tumors, and spontaneous pneumothorax. Fibrofolliculomas are part of the triad of BHD skin lesions that also includes trichodiscomas and acrochordons. Onset of this dermatologic condition is invariably in adulthood. BHD is associated with a variety of histologic types of renal tumors, including chromophobe renal cell carcinoma (RCC), benign renal oncocytoma, clear-cell RCC and papillary type I RCC. Multiple lipomas,

angiolipomas, and parathyroid adenomas are also seen in patients affected with this disease. The majority of mutations are predicted to prematurely terminate the protein.
- BHD syndrome is characterized by a spectrum of mutations (at least 23 different germline mutations, of various types), and clinical heterogeneity both among and within families. All germline mutations are predicted to truncate the mutant protein. Mutations are located along the entire length of the coding region, with no genotype-phenotype correlations noted between type of mutation, location within the gene and phenotypic disease manifestations. More than 50% of mutations have been observed in a hotspot in exon 11
- FLCN somatic mutations have been found at only a very low frequency (0-10%) in sporadic renal tumors and therefore, may not represent a major mechanism for the development of sporadic renal carcinoma. Loss of 17p DNA including p53 or partial methylation of the FLCN promoter were reported in sporadic renal carcinomas with various histologies.
- Mutations have been identified in the mutational hotspot in exon 11 of FLCN in other tumor types exhibiting microsatellite instability, including colorectal carcinoma (20%), endometrial carcinoma (12%) and gastric carcinoma (16%).

FLT3 (13q12)
Fms-Related Tyrosine Kinase 3

Function

FLT3 (Langdon 2012) encodes a protein tyrosine kinase receptor for the FL cytokine. FL is an early acting factor and supports the survival, proliferation and differentiation of primitive hemopoietic progenitor cells.

Ligand binding to FLT3 promotes receptor dimerization and subsequent signaling through phosphorylation of multiple cytoplasmatic proteins, including SHC, SHP-2, SHIP, Cbl, Cbl-b, Gab1 and Gab2, as well as the activation of several downstream signaling pathways, such as the Ras/Raf/MAPK and PI3 kinase cascades.

Cancer-Related Gene Alterations

- Somatic mutations in the FLT3 gene are the most frequent genetic aberration that have been described in acute myeloid leukemia. Mutations have also been observed in bile duct tumors. These somatic mutations are highly frequent in two regions corresponding to amino acids 550-650 and 831-842. In this latter region, corresponding to the second tyrosine kinase kinase domain of FLT3, alterations are mostly point mutations related to codon 835 or deletions related to codon 836. These mutations lead to constitutive autoactivation of the receptor.
- FLT3-length mutations (FLT3-LM), in which internal tandem duplications and/or insertions and, rarely, deletions in the FLT3-gene occur, are implicated in 20-25% of all acute myeloid leukemias. They were also described to be involved in 5-10 % myelodysplastic syndromes, refractory anemia with excess of blasts and rare cases with acute lymphoblastic leukemia.

In FLT3-LM, mutations lead to constitutive ligand independent autophosphorylation of the receptor.

The duplicated sequence belongs to exon 11 but sometimes involves intron 11 and exon 12. FLT3-LM are highly correlated with a) normal karyotype, b) t(15;17)(q25;q21) translocation.

FOXL2 (3q23)
Forkhead Box L2

Function
FOXL2 (Verdin and De Baere 2012) encodes a transcription factor with a fork-head DNA-binding domain.

FOXL2 is a critical factor essential for ovary differentiation and maintenance, and repression of the genetic program for somatic testis determination.

Prevents trans-differentiation of ovary to testis through transcriptional repression of the Sertoli cell-promoting gene SOX9 and may play a role in ovarian development and function.

Cancer-Related Gene Alterations
- Somatic mutations, consisting in substitutions only, are observed in about 25% of ovarian cancers. More than 95% of mutations target amino acid 134.

GATA1 (Xp11.23)
GATA Binding Protein 1 (Globin Transcription Factor 1)

Function
GATA1 (Crispino 2005) encodes a protein which belongs to the GATA family of transcription factors. GATA1 is essential for erythroid and megakaryocytic development. It helps transcribe the α-spectrin structural protein which is critical for the shape of red blood cells.

Cancer-Related Gene Alterations
- Somatic mutations are seen in hematopoietic and lymphoid tissue tumors. They alter the first 80 amino acids of the protein.
- Acquired somatic mutations in GATA1 occur in virtually all children with Down Syndrome (DS) and congenital transient myeloproliferative syndrome (TMD) or acute megakaryocytic leukemia (AMKL).

  The mutations have also been detected in umbilical cord blood of DS patients and in fetal liver of aborted DS embryos. These mutations occur *in-utero* probably during fetal liver hematopoiesis.

  They consist of insertions, deletions and base substitution in exon 2 and vicinity and all result in elimination of the full length GATA1 protein with preservation of the GATA1 isoforms.

GATA3 (10p15)
GATA Binding Protein 3

Function
GATA3 (Chou et al. 2010) encodes a protein which belongs to the GATA family of transcription factors. The protein is an important regulator of T-cell development and plays an important role in endothelial cell biology. GATA3 regulates estrogen receptor expression in breast cancer.

Cancer-Related Gene Alterations
- Somatic mutations (deletions, insertions, substitutions) have been observed in tumors of breast (>10%) and large intestine (>10%). Most insertions and deletions are seen in the C-terminal (amino acids 300-445) of the protein.

GNAQ (9q21)
Guanine Nucleotide Binding Protein (G Protein), Q Polypeptide

Function
GNAQ (Sisley et al. 2011) encodes a heterotrimeric GTP-binding protein α-subunit that couples G-protein coupled receptor signaling to the MAP kinase pathway. GNAQ codon 209 mutations form an alternative route to MAP kinase activation. GNAQ is important in melanocyte homeostasis and survival of melanocytes early in neural crest development.

Cancer-Related Gene Alterations
- Frequent somatic mutations have recently been identified in the ras-like domain of GNAQ in blue naevi (83%), malignant blue naevi (50%) and ocular melanoma of the uvea (46%). The mutations exclusively affect codon 209, prevent hydrolysis of GTP and turns GNAQ into its active, GTP-bound state. It results the constitutive activation of GNAQ. Thus, GNAQ acts as a dominant oncogene.
- Somatic mutations in the GNAQ gene at codon 209 are a frequent event in primary melanocytic neoplasms of the CNS. More than 99% of these mutations are substitutions missense.

GNAS (20q13.32)
GNAS Complex Locus

Function
GNAS (Weinstein et al. 2004) generates multiple gene products through the use of alternative promoters and first exons that splice onto a common exon. The most downstream alternative promoter generates transcripts encoding the ubiquitously expressed G protein α-subunit Gsα that couples many receptors for hormones, neurotransmitters and other extracellular signals to adenylyl cyclase. Gsα is required for receptor-stimulated cAMP production and most of its downstream effects are mediated via cAMP, which in turn activates signaling molecules such as protein kinase A (PKA) and cAMP-regulated guanine

nucleotide exchange factors (cAMP-GEFs). PKA acutely activates many metabolic processes such as lipolysis, gluconeogenesis, and glycogenolysis.

Cancer-Related Gene Alterations
- GNAS mutations result in various non-cancerous diseases: pseudohypoparathyroidism type 1a, pseudohypoparathyroidism type 1b, Albright hereditary osteodystrophy, pseudopseudohypoparathyroidism, McCune-Albright syndrome, progressive osseous heteroplasia, polyostotic fibrous dysplasia of bone. Genetic alterations in GNAS may also be the cause of a subset of growth hormone secreting pituitary tumors (somatotrophinoma).
- Somatic GNAS point mutations (exclusively substitution missense) have been observed in tumors of pituitary (about 25% of cases), ovary and testis (about 15%) parathyroid, kidney, thyroid, adrenal gland, large intestine, autonomic ganglia and lung.
- There are two mutation hotspots corresponding to amino acids 201 and 227.

HNF1A (12q24.2)
HNF1 Homeobox A

Function

HNF1A (Armendariz and Krauss 2009) encodes a transcriptional activator that functions as a homodimer and regulates the tissue specific expression of multiple genes, especially in pancreatic islet cells and in liver.

Cancer-Related Gene Alterations
- Defects in HNF1A are a cause of hepatic adenomas familial (HEPAF). Hepatic adenomas are rare benign liver tumors of presumable epithelial origin that develop in an otherwise normal liver. Hepatic adenomas may be single or multiple. They consist of sheets of well-differentiated hepatocytes that contain fat and glycogen and can produce bile. Bile ducts or portal areas are absent. If present, Kupffer cells are reduced in number and are non-functional. Conditions associated with adenomas are insulin-dependent diabetes mellitus and glycogen storage diseases (types 1 and 3).
- Somatic HNF1A mutations (deletions, insertions, substitutions…) have been observed in liver (about 20% of cases), large intestine, endometrium and breast tumors. Mutation distribution is variable, with, however, amino acids 291 and 292 as hot spots for deletions and insertions, respectively.

HRAS (11p15.5)
v-Ha-ras Harvey Rat Sarcoma Viral Oncogene Homolog

Function

The protein encoded by this gene (Baines et al. 2011) belongs to the Ras oncogene family, whose members are related to the transforming genes of mammalian sarcoma retroviruses. The products encoded by these genes function in signal transduction pathways.

These proteins can bind GTP and GDP, and they have intrinsic GTPase activity. This protein undergoes a continuous cycle of de- and re-palmitoylation, which regulates its rapid exchange between the plasma membrane and the Golgi apparatus.

Cancer-Related Gene Alterations
- Somatic HRAS mutations have been observed in tumors of salivary glands (about 15% of cases), urinary tract, upper aerodigestive tract (oral squamous cell carcinoma) and cervix. In most cases, mutations are substitution missenses. Mutation hotspots are related to amino acids 12, 13 and 61. HRAS-associated bladder cancer often presents with multiple tumors appearing at different times and at different sites in the bladder.
- HRAS mutations may be the cause of Costello syndrome, a disease characterized by increased growth at the prenatal stage, growth deficiency at the postnatal stage, predisposition to tumor formation, mental retardation, skin and musculoskeletal abnormalities, distinctive facial appearance and cardiovascular abnormalities. Defects in HRAS are the cause of congenital myopathy with excess of muscle spindles (CMEMS), which is a variant of Costello syndrome.
- Hurthle cell thyroid carcinoma, which accounts for approximately 3% of all thyroid cancers, is associated to HRAS genetic alterations. Although Hurthle cell thyroid carcinomas are classified as variants of follicular neoplasms, they are more often multifocal and somewhat more aggressive and are less likely to take up iodine than are other follicular neoplasms.

IDH1 (2q33.3) and **IDH2** (15q26.1)
Isocitrate Dehydrogenase 1 (NADP+), Soluble and Isocitrate Dehydrogenase 2 (NADP+), Mitochondrial

Function

Isocitrate dehydrogenases (Borodovsky et al. 2012) catalyze the oxidative decarboxylation of isocitrate to 2-oxoglutarate. IDH1 localizes to the cytoplasm and peroxisomes, and acts as a NADP-dependent protein that catalyzes decarboxylation of isocitrate into α-ketoglutarate. IDH2 is the only protein homologous to IDH1 that also utilizes NADP; however IDH2 localizes to the mitochondria.

IDH2 plays an important role in controlling the mitochondrial redox balance, and in providing protection from oxidative damage similar to IDH1.

Cancer-Related Gene Alterations
- Genetic alterations in IDH1 or IDH2 have been found in malignant brain tumors. While IDH1 or IDH2 mutations are observed in the majority of grade II and III astrocytomas and oligodendrogliomas, glioblastomas and low grade astrocytic tumors demonstrate an absence or low frequency of mutations. All IDH alterations are point mutations resulting in a missense change at codon 132 of IDH1, and codons 140 or 172 of IDH2. Residues 132 of IDH1 and 172 of IDH2 are analogous between genes, and occur in exon 4 at a highly conserved region of the isocitrate binding site.

The mutation is thought to down-regulate or even eliminate enzyme activity, leading to increased cellular oxidative stress and damage.
- IDH1 or IDH2 mutations have also been observed in about 10% of AML cases.

JAK2 (9p24)
Janus kinase 2

Function
Janus tyrosine kinase 2 (Jak2), the protein coded by JAK2, is a protein tyrosine kinase of the non-receptor type that associates with the intracellular domains of various receptors. It plays pivotal functions for signal transduction from hematopoietic cytokine (IL-3, GM-CSF, and erythropoietin) receptors, mediating the activation of STAT proteins, required in definitive erythropoiesis.

Jak2 is also involved in growth hormone (GH) induced activation of the GH receptor. It has been found to be constitutively associated with the prolactin receptor.

Cancer-Related Gene Alterations
- Four translocations involving JAK2 have been described to date:
  - t(5;9)(q14.1;p24.1), leading to SSBP2-JAK2, is observed in pre-B-ALL
  - t(8;9)(p22;p24), leading to PCM1-JAK2, is observed in atypical CML, chronic eosinophilic leukemia (CEL), ALL and NHL
  - t(9;12)(p24;p13), leading to JAK2-ETV6, is observed in T-ALL, B-ALL, CML
  - t(9;22)(p24;q11.2), leading to JAK2-BCR, is observed in CML B-ALL: B-cell acute lymphocytic leukemia; T-ALL: T-cell acute lymphocytic leukemia;
- Somatic JAK2 mutations are seen in about 40% of hematopoietic and lymphoid tissue tumors. More than 50% of patients with myeloproliferative disorders (MPD) (polycythemia vera, essential thrombocythemia, idiopathic myelofibrosis) carry a dominant gain-of-function V617F mutation in the "JH2 kinase-like" domain of JAK2.

This mutation leads to deregulation of the kinase activity, and thus to constitutive tyrosine phosphorylation activity.

In MPD the mutation is heterozygous in most patients and homozygous only in a minor subset. Mitotic recombination probably causes both 9p LOH and the transition from heterozygosity to homozygosity.

The same mutation was also found in roughly 20% of "Philadelphia Chromosome negative" (Ph-negative) atypical CML, in more than 10% of chronic myelomonocytic leukemia (CMML), in about 15% of patients with megakaryocytic AML, and 1 of 5 patients with juvenile myelomonocytic leukemia.

The V617F mutation seems to occur exclusively in hematopoietic malignancies of the myeloid lineage (Oh and Gotlib 2010).

KIT (4q12)
v-kit Hardy-Zuckerman 4 Feline Sarcoma Viral Oncogene Homolog

Function

KIT encodes the receptor for stem cell factor. It is a tyrosine-protein kinase activity. Binding of the ligands leads to the autophosphorylation of KIT and its association with substrates such as phosphatidylinositol 3-kinase (Pi3K).

Cancer-Related Gene Alterations
- Germinal KIT mutations are a cause of familial GISTs (Fletcher and Rubin 2007). GISTs are the most common mesenchymal tumors in the human digestive tract; they originate from KIT-expressing cells and often have activating KIT mutations clustered in the juxtamembrane domain. GISTs may also be caused by somatic KIT alterations. Mutations in PDGFRA may also induce GISTs.
- Somatic KIT mutations are observed in many tumor types. These include tumors of soft tissue, hematopoietic and lymphoid tissue, genital tract, testis, salivary glands… KIT mutations are notably involved in systemic mast cell disease (SMCD), which is characterized by cell hyperplasia in the bone marrow, liver, spleen, lymph nodes, gastrointestinal tract and skin; gain of function mutations are detected in most patients.
- KIT mutations are also seen in core binding factor (CBF) leukemias, which are characterized by disruption and loss of CBFa2/AML1 - CBFb/PEBP2b function.
- Substitutions account for about one-half of somatic mutations. There is a mutation hot spot corresponding to amino acid 816 and around this site. Most complex mutations are seen in regions corresponding to amino acids 417-419 and 547-571.

KLF6 (10p15)
Kruppel-Like Factor 6

Function

This gene (Narla et al. 2003) encodes a member of the Kruppel-like factor family of transcriptional regulators involved in development and differentiation as well as in growth signaling pathways, apoptosis, proliferation and angiogenesis. KLF6 functions as a tumor suppressor.

Multiple transcript variants encoding different isoforms have been found for this gene, some of which are implicated in carcinogenesis.

Cancer-Related Gene Alterations
- Somatic KLF6 mutations have been reported in astrocytoma, glioblastoma and meningioma, nasopharyngeal carcinoma, prostate cancer, colorectal cancer, hepatocellular carcinoma, gastric cancer. Most mutation events are substitutions.

KRAS (12p12.1)
v-Ki-ras2 Kirsten Rat Sarcoma Viral Oncogene Homolog

Function

This gene, a Kirsten ras oncogene homolog from the mammalian ras gene family, encodes a protein that is a member of the small GTPase superfamily. It plays a crucial role in signal transduction in many tissues.

Cancer-Related Gene Alterations
- KRAS (Baines et al. 2011) is one of the most frequently mutated genes in a variety of tumors. Most alterations are missense substitutions. There are three mutation hot spots, corresponding to amino acids 12, 13 and 61. A majority of oncogenic KRAS proteins have impaired intrinsic and GAP-mediated GTP hydrolysis and thus express constitutive GTP-bound activity.
- Somatic KRAS mutations are common in tumors of the following tissues: pancreas (more than 50% of cases), large intestine, biliary tract, small intestine, lung, endometrium and ovary.

MAP2K4 (17p11.2)
Mitogen-Activated Protein Kinase Kinase 4 (Also Known as MKK4)

Function

This gene encodes a dual specificity protein kinase (Cuenda 2000) that belongs to the serine/threonine protein kinase family. This kinase is a direct activator of MAP kinases in response to various environmental stresses or mitogenic stimuli. It has been shown to activate MAPK8 (also known as JNK1), MAPK9 (JNK2), and MAPK14 (p38), but not MAPK1 (ERK2) or MAPK3 (ERK3). This kinase is phosphorylated, and thus activated by MAP3K1 (MEKK). The knockout studies in mice suggested the roles of this kinase in mediating survival signal in T cell development, as well as in the organogenesis of liver.

Cancer-Related Gene Alterations
- Somatic MAP2K4 mutations (of which 40% are substitutions) have been found in tumors of endometrium (about 10% of cases), pancreas, breast, large intestine, biliary tract, testis, urinary tract.

MAP3K1 (5q11.2)
Mitogen-Activated Protein Kinase Kinase Kinase 1, E3 Ubiquitin Protein Ligase

Function

This gene (Stephens et al. 2010) encodes a serine/threonine protein kinase that is part of some signal transduction cascades, including the ERK and JNK kinase pathways as well as the NFκB pathway. Activation of the ERK and JNK kinase pathways is notably mediated by phosphorylation of MAP2K4.

Cancer-related gene alterations
- Somatic MAP3K1 mutations (of which 75% are substitutions) have been found in tumors of large intestine (10%) and breast (about 2% of cases).

MAP3K13 (3q27.2)
Mitogen-Activated Protein Kinase Kinase Kinase 13

Function

This gene (Stephens et al. 2010) encodes a serine/threonine protein kinase that activates the JUN N-terminal pathway through activation of MAP2K7 (also known as MKK7). It also activates MAPK8 (JNK1). MAP3K13 acts synergistically with the mitochondrial thioredoxin-dependent peroxide reductase (PRDX3) to regulate the activation of NF-kappa-B in the cytosol.

Cancer-Related Gene Alterations
- Somatic MAP3K13 mutations (of which a majority are missense substitutions) have been found in tumors of large intestine (>10%), breast (>10%), and ovary (>5%). No mutation hot spot has been identified.

MEN1 (11q13.1)
Multiple Endocrine Neoplasia I

Function

MEN1 product, menin (Balogh et al. 2010), is a growth-suppressor gene. It interacts with the AP1 transcription factor through his JunD component, but with none of the other AP1 proteins, such as JunB, c-Jun, c-Fos and Fra1/2. Many cellular functions of menin have been identified. However, it remains unclear which ones of these relate specifically to menin's role as a tumor suppressor and which ones not. Menin is predominantly nuclear and acts as a scaffold protein to regulate gene transcription by coordinating chromatin remodeling. It is implicated in both histone deacetylase and histone methyltransferase activity and, via the latter, regulates the expression of cell cycle kinase inhibitor and homeobox domain genes. TGF-β family members are key cytostatic molecules and menin is a facilitator of the transcriptional activity of their signaling molecules, the Smads, thereby ensuring appropriate control of cell proliferation and differentiation

Cancer-Related Gene Alterations
- Germline mutations in the MEN1 gene cause familial and sporadic multiple endocrine neoplasia type 1 (MEN1). Familial MEN1 is an autosomal dominant disorder characterized by a predisposition to endocrine tumors, including parathyroid, gastrointestinal endocrine tissue, endocrine pancreas, pituitary, adrenal glands, thymus… The majority of mutations described predict premature protein truncation either by nonsenses and frameshifts in coding sequences, but missense mutations have also been identified in about 30% of cases.

- Between 10 and 15% of sporadic MEN1 could be explained by *de novo* mutations.
- Approximately 10-15% of MEN1 families do not show any mutation in the known part of MEN1 sequence; clinical profile in these families do not differ from that of families with identified mutations and it is therefore possible that MEN1 mutations occur outside the coding sequence
- Prognosis in MEN1 patients is mainly related to metabolic and organic complications of hormonal hypersecretion by tumoral cells, such as hypergastrinemia causing severe peptic ulcer disease (Zollinger-Ellison syndrome), primary hyperparathyroidism, and acute forms of hyperinsulinemia.
- It seems that some MEN1 families could express only primary hyperparathyroidism, so called familial primary hyperparathyroidism (FIHPT), an allelic variant of MEN1. FIHPT is an autosomal dominant disorder characterized by hypercalcemia, elevated parathyroid hormone (PTH) levels, and uniglandular or multiglandular parathyroid tumors.

MLH1 (3p21.3) and **MSH2** (2p22-p21) and **MSH6** (2p16)
Mutl Homolog 1, Colon Cancer, Nonpolyposis Type 2 (E. Coli) and Muts Homolog 2, Colon Cancer, Nonpolyposis Type 1 (E. Coli) and Muts Homolog 6 (E. Coli)

Function

MLH1 forms heterodimer with PMS2 (MutLα), PMS1 (MutLβ) or MLH3 (MutLγ). MutLα is a component of the post-replicative DNA mismatch repair system (MMR). DNA repair is initiated by MutSα (MSH2-MSH6) or MutSβ (MSH2-MSH3), which recognize and bind to a dsDNA mismatch, then MutLα is recruited to the heteroduplex. While MutSα complex binds to base-base and insertion-deletion mismatches, MutSβ only binds to insertion-deletion mismatches. Assembly of the MutL-MutS-heteroduplex ternary complex in presence of RFC (replication factor C) and PCNA (Proliferating Cell Nuclear Antigen) is sufficient to activate endonuclease activity of PMS2 (it seems that MLH1 itself has no enzymatic activity). It introduces single-strand breaks near the mismatch and thus generates new entry points for the exonuclease EXO1 to degrade the strand containing the mismatch. DNA methylation would prevent cleavage and therefore assure that only the newly mutated DNA strand is going to be corrected. MutLα interacts physically with the clamp loader subunits of DNA polymerase III, suggesting that it may play a role to recruit the DNA polymerase III to the site of the MMR. In fact, MutLα is thought to be responsible for directing the downstream MMR events, including strand discrimination, excision, and resynthesis. Also implicated in DNA damage signaling, a process which induces cell cycle arrest and can lead to apoptosis in case of major DNA damages.

MLH1, MSH2 and MSH6 (Marti et al. 2002) are part of the BRCA1-associated genome surveillance complex (BASC), which contains BRCA1, MSH2, MSH6, MLH1, ATM, BLM, PMS2 and the RAD50-MRE11-NBS1 protein complex. This association could be a dynamic process changing throughout the cell cycle and within subnuclear domains.

Cancer-Related Gene Alterations

- Defects in a) MLH1, b) MSH2 and c) MSH6 are the cause of a) hereditary non-polyposis colorectal cancer type 2 (HNPCC2), b) HNPCC1 (and HNPCC8, see below) and c) HNPCC5, respectively. Mutations in more than one gene locus can be involved alone or in combination in the production of the HNPCC phenotype (also called Lynch syndrome). Most families with clinically recognized HNPCC have mutations in either MLH1 or MSH2 genes (25% of cases each). HNPCC is an autosomal, dominantly inherited disease associated with marked increase in cancer susceptibility. It is characterized by a familial predisposition to early onset colorectal carcinoma (CRC) and extra-colonic cancers of the gastrointestinal, urological and female reproductive tracts. HNPCC is reported to be the most common form of inherited colorectal cancer in the Western world, and accounts for 15% of all colon cancers. Cancers in HNPCC originate within benign neoplastic polyps termed adenomas.

Clinically, HNPCC is often divided into two subgroups:

- Type I: hereditary predisposition to colorectal cancer, a young age of onset, and carcinoma observed in the proximal colon.
- Type II: patients have an increased risk for cancers in certain tissues such as the uterus, ovary, breast, stomach, small intestine, skin, and larynx in addition to the colon.

Diagnosis of classical HNPCC is based on the Amsterdam criteria:

- 3 or more relatives affected by colorectal cancer, one a first degree relative of the other two;
- 2 or more generation affected;
- 1 or more colorectal cancers presenting before 50 years of age; exclusion of hereditary polyposis syndromes.

MSH6 mutations (10% of HNPCC cases) appear to be associated with atypical HNPCC and in particular with development of endometrial carcinoma or atypical endometrial hyperplasia, the presumed precursor of endometrial cancer. Defects in MSH6 are also found in familial colorectal cancers (suspected or incomplete HNPCC) that do not fulfill the Amsterdam criteria for HNPCC.

Defects in MSH2 are a cause of a particular type of HNPCC named HNPCC8, resulting from heterozygous deletion of 3-prime exons of EPCAM and intergenic regions directly upstream of MSH2; the consequence is a read-through and epigenetic silencing of MSH2 in tissues expressing EPCAM.

- Germinal mutations: there are over 300 MLH1 and 300 MSH2 germline mutations described that cause HNPCC. These mutations are not present in any particular hotspot or zone of the gene and include either nucleotide substitutions (missense, nonsense or splicing errors) or insertions/deletions (gross or small). In most cases, the resulting protein is truncated. There are also founding mutations which account

for a high proportion of the HNPCC tumors in some specific populations (for example there are two Finnish mutations that delete the exons 16 or 6). Regarding MSH6, its germline mutations have variable penetration and are relatively rare in HNPCC and HNPCC-like families.
- Somatic ML1, MSH2 and MSH6 mutations have been observed mainly in tumors of large intestine, stomach, ovary and endometrium. These mutations are not present in any particular hot spot or zone of the gene and include either nucleotide substitutions (missense, nonsense or splicing errors) or insertions/deletions (gross or small). Somatic MLH1 and MSH2 mutation may cause microsatellite instability (MSI) in colorectal, gastric and endometrial cancer. The involvement of somatic or epigenetic inactivation of MSH6 is rare in colorectal cancer and missense mutations in MSH6 are often clinically innocuous or have a low penetrance. However, somatic mutations of MSH6 have been shown to confer resistance to alkylating agents such as temozolomide in malignant gliomas *in vivo*.
- Microsatellite instability (MSI) is a characteristic of tumors in which the molecular feature that leads to cancer is the lost of the mismatch repair (MMR) system. This phenotype is present in 15% of colorectal, gastric and endometrial cancer, and with lower incidence in some other tissues. MSI may be due to sporadic or germline (in HNPCC) mutations in MLH1 or MSH2.
- Germline alterations in MLH1 or MSH2 are a cause of Muir-Torre syndrome (MuToS). MuToS is a rare autosomal dominant disorder characterized by sebaceous neoplasms and visceral malignancy.
- Defects in MLH1 or MSH6 are a cause of mismatch repair cancer syndrome (MMRCS) MMRCS is an autosomal dominant disorder characterized by malignant tumors of the brain associated with multiple colorectal adenomas. Skin features include sebaceous cysts, hyperpigmented and café-au-lait spots. MSH2 mutations may predispose to hematological malignancies and multiple café-au-lait spots.

MPL (1p34)
Myeloproliferative Leukemia Virus Oncogene

Function
The protein encoded by MPL (Chou and Mulloy 2010) is a receptor for thrombopoietin (TPO-R). Thrombopoietin is the major regulator of megakaryocytopoiesis and platelet formation. Upon binding of thrombopoietin, TPO-R is dimerized and the JAK family of non-receptor tyrosine kinases, as well as the STAT family, the MAPK family, the adaptor protein Shc and the receptors themselves become tyrosine phosphorylated.

Cancer-Related Gene Alterations
- Somatic MPL mutations (essentially missense substitutions) have been found exclusively in hematopoietic and lymphoid tissue tumors. These mutations are observed in a region corresponding to amino acids 505-519, with a hotspot at amino acid 515

MUTYH (1p34.1)
MutY homolog (E. coli)

Function

MUTYH (Zorcolo et al. 2011) encodes a DNA glycosylase involved in oxidative DNA damage repair. The enzyme excises adenine bases from the DNA backbone at sites where adenine is inappropriately paired with guanine, cytosine, or 8-oxo-7,8-dihydroguanine, a major oxidatively damaged DNA lesion. MUTYH functions in a postreplication repair pathway and is targeted to the newly synthesized daughter strand of DNA for removal of the adenine base.

Cancer-Related Gene Alterations
- Biallelic MUTYH germline mutations are associated with the autosomal recessive form of intestinal adenomatous polyposis (MUTYH-associated polyposis, or MAP). The most common mutations in Caucasians are the missense substitutions Y165C and G382D. Functional analysis of C165 and D382 proteins has shown a severe decrease of catalytic activity. E466X and Y90X are the common mutations reported in Indian and Pakistani cases. Several other missense, nonsense, in-frame, frameshift and splicing mutations have been found in patients with MAP. Defective base excision repair function associated with MUTYH mutations determines an increase in the somatic mutation rate. Tumors from biallelic MUTYH mutation carriers display an excess of somatic G>T mutations in the APC and KRAS genes.
- To date, no somatic MUTYH mutation has been described.

MYC (8q24.21)
v-myc Myelocytomatosis Viral Oncogene Homolog (Avian)

Function

The protein encoded by this gene (Dang 2010) is a multifunctional phosphoprotein that plays a role in cell cycle progression, apoptosis and cellular transformation. It functions as a transcription factor that regulates the expression of specific target genes. Binding of Myc requires dimerization to another protein, namely Max. Myc/Max complexes activate transcription and promote cell proliferation and transformation. Expression of Myc is required for proliferation.

Cancer-Related Gene Alterations
- Genetic alterations of MYC are implicated in the etiology of a variety of tumors, including breast, cervical and colon cancers, as well as in squamous cell carcinomas of the head and neck, myeloma, non-Hodgkin's lymphoma, gastric adenocarcinomas and ovarian cancer. MYC gene activation (enhanced expression and/or amplification) may result from chromosomal duplication as well as translocation, and from retroviral as well as point mutation.
- Genetic alterations involving MYC are a cause of Burkitt lymphoma (BL), a form of undifferentiated malignant lymphoma commonly manifested as a large osteolytic lesion in the jaw or as an abdominal mass. Translocations t(2;8)(p11;q24),

t(8;14)(q24;q32) or t(8;22)(q24;q11) juxtaposing MYC to immunoglobin chains IGK@, IGH@ or IGL@, respectively, are usually found in Burkitt lymphoma.
- Translocations may also lead to BCL6-MYC (t(3;8)(q27;q24.1)), MYC-ZBTB5 (t(8;9)(q24;p13)), MYC-ZCCHC7 (t(8;9)(q24;p13)), BTG1-MYC (t(8;12)(q21;q22)), TRA@-MYC (t(8;14)(q24;q11)), MYC-BCL3 (t(8;19)(q24;q13.1)) in NHL, CLL, B-ALL and AML.

NCOR1 (17p11.2)
Nuclear receptor corepressor 1

Function
NCOR1 encodes a transcriptional repressor of certain nuclear receptors (Battaglia et al. 2010). It is part of a complex which promotes histone acetylation and the formation of repressive chromatin structures which may impede the access of basal transcription factors.

Cancer-Related Gene Alterations
- Somatic NCOR1 mutations are mainly substitutions. They are found in tumors of breast (>30%), large intestine (>30%) and upper aerodigestive tract (>60%).

NF1 (17q12) and NF2 (22q12.2)
Neurofibromin 1 and Neurofibromin 2 (Merlin)

Function
NF1 encodes neurofibromin (Yohay 2006), a protein that is produced in many types of cells, including nerve cells and specialized cells called oligodendrocytes and Schwann cells that surround nerves. These specialized cells form myelin sheaths, which are the fatty coverings that insulate and protect certain nerve cells. Neurofibromin acts as a tumor suppressor protein. It prevents cell overgrowth by turning off the ras signal transduction pathway that stimulates cell growth and division.

The product of NF2 gene (Yohay 2006) is merlin (moesin-ezrin-radixin-like protein). It is a multifunctional protein involved in integrating and regulating the extracellular cues and intracellular signaling pathways that control cell fate, shape, proliferation, survival, and motility. In adults, significant NF2 expression is found in Schwann cells, meningeal cells, lens and nerve.

Cancer-related Gene Alterations
- Germinal mutations: large NF1 submicroscopic deletions are observed in 5-10% of cases, translocations are rare and point mutations are seen in approximately 85-90% of cases; mutations are widely dispersed, with no clustering, and unusual splicing mutations yield difficulties in molecular genetic testing. Mutations have a truncating effect in a large majority of cases.
NF2 protein truncations are frequently observed, due to various frameshift deletions or insertions or nonsense mutations; splice-site or missense mutations are also found;

phenotype-genotype correlations are observed (i.e. severe phenotypes are found in cases with protein truncations rather than those with amino acid substitution)
- Somatic mutations: NF1 and NF2 somatic mutations have been identified in tumors of soft tissues, thyroid, stomach, CNS, skin...NF1 mutations have also been observed in colorectal and autonomic ganglia (ganglioneuromas) tumors. NF2 somatic mutations have also been found in tumors of meninges (meningioma), pleura (mesothelioma), urinary tract and endometrium. These mutations are various (deletions, insertions, point mutations). There are no mutation hotspots in NF1; in NF2, two substitution hotspots correspond to amino acids 57 and 341.
- Defects in NF1 are the cause of type 1 neurofibromatosis (NF1). NF1 is one of the most frequent autosomal dominant diseases (about 1 in 3000 births). It exhibits full penetrance by the age of 5 years and high mutation rate with 30 to 50% of NF1 patients representing a new mutation. Among the many clinical features of NF1 are patches of skin pigmentation (café-au-lait spots), Lisch nodules of the iris, peripheral nervous system associated tumors and fibromatous skin tumors.
- Defects in NF1 are the cause of Watson syndrome (WS), which is an autosomal dominant disease with cardiac malformations pulmonary stenosis, cafe-au-lait spots, and mental retardation. WS is considered as an atypical form of NF1.
- Defects in NF1 are a cause of JMML, a pediatric myelodysplastic syndrome (MDS) that constitutes approximately 30% of childhood cases of MDS and 2% of leukemia. Germline mutations of NF1 account for the association of JMML with type 1 neurofibromatosis (NF1).
- Defects in NF1 are a cause of familial spinal neurofibromatosis (spinal NF). Familial spinal NF is considered to be an alternative form of neurofibromatosis, showing multiple spinal tumors.
- Defects in NF1 are a cause of neurofibromatosis-Noonan syndrome (NFNS). NFNS is characterized by manifestations of both NF1 and Noonan syndrome (NS). NS is a disorder characterized by dysmorphic facial features, short stature, hypertelorism, cardiac anomalies, deafness, motor delay, and a bleeding diathesis.
- Defects in NF2 are the cause of type II neurofibromatosis (NF2). NF2 is a genetic disorder characterized by bilateral vestibular schwannomas (formerly called acoustic neuromas), schwannomas of other cranial and peripheral nerves, meningiomas, and ependymomas. Skin tumors and ocular abnormalities are also observed. It is inherited in an autosomal dominant fashion with full penetrance. Affected individuals generally develop symptoms of eighth-nerve dysfunction in early adulthood, including deafness and balance disorder. Although the tumors of NF2 are histologically benign, their anatomic location makes management difficult, and patients suffer great morbidity and mortality.
- Defects in NF2 are a cause of schwannomatosis; also known as congenital cutaneous neurilemmomatosis. Schwannomas are benign tumors of the peripheral nerve sheath that usually occur singly in otherwise normal individuals. Multiple schwannomas in the same individual suggest an underlying tumor-predisposition syndrome. The most common such syndrome is NF2. The hallmark of NF2 is the development of bilateral vestibular-nerve schwannomas; but two-thirds or more of all NF2-affected individuals develop schwannomas in other locations, and dermal schwannomas may precede vestibular tumors in NF2-affected children. There have been several reports

of individuals with multiple schwannomas who do not show evidence of vestibular schwannoma. Clinical report suggests that schwannomatosis is a clinical entity distinct from other forms of neurofibromatosis.

NOTCH1 (9q34.3)
Notch 1

Function
The protein encoded by NOTCH1 functions as a receptor for membrane-bound ligands of the Jagged and Delta-like families. It is involved in cell-fate determination, implementation of differentiation, proliferation and apoptotic programs.

Cancer-Related Gene Alterations
- NOTCH1 (Palomero and Ferrando 2008) play a dual role in carcinogenesis as either a tumor suppressor or an oncogene. The role of NOTCH1 within and between cells depends on signal strength, timing, cell type, and context.
- Altered NOTCH1 is a causative factor in the development of T-ALL. It is notably involved in T-ALL following translocation t(7;9)(q34;q34.3), leading to the fusion gene NOTCH1-TRB@, in which the 3' portion of NOTCH1 is juxtaposed with the T cell receptor β (TRB@) locus. This leads to expression of truncated NOTCH1 transcripts and consequent production of dominant active, ligand-independent forms of the NOTCH1 receptor, causing T-ALL. Less than 1% of human T-ALL exhibit the t(7;9) translocation, however, activating mutations in NOTCH1 independent of t(7;9) have been identified in more than 50% of human T-ALL.
- Somatic point mutations have been found in tumors of hematopoietic and lymphoid tissue (up to 20%), esophagus and upper aerodigestive tract, CNS, large intestine, lung, pancreas, breast. Most mutation events are substitution, with hotspots corresponding to amino acids 1575-1601.

NPM1 (5q35.1)
Nucleophosmin

Function
NPM1 (Falini et al. 2011) encodes a phosphoprotein involved in diverse cellular processes such as ribosome biogenesis, centrosome duplication, protein chaperoning, histone assembly, cell proliferation, and regulation of tumor suppressors p53 (gene TP53) and p16^{INK4} (gene CDKN2A). NPM1 protein binds ribosome presumably to drive ribosome nuclear export. It associates with nucleolar ribonucleoprotein structures and bind single-stranded nucleic acids. It acts as a chaperonin for the core histones H3, H2B and H4.

Cancer-Related Gene Alterations
- NPM1 somatic mutations have been observed in hematopoietic/lymphoid tissue and in bile duct tumors. Mutations in the form of nucleotide insertions in exon 12 of NPM1 are found in 25-35% of all cases of acute myeloid leukemia (AML). Most

NPM1 mutations occur in exon 12. They generate an extra nuclear export signal motif and cause loss of tryptophan 288 and 290 (or tryptophan 290 alone); as a result, NPM1 accumulates aberrantly in the cytoplasm. Because NPM1 is thought to possess a tumor-suppressor function, any disruption in its cellular localization may be critical for malignant transformation.

- NPM1 is involved in fusions with ALK in anaplasic large cell lymphoma (ALCL), a form of high-grade non-Hodgkin lymphoma. Translocation t(2;5)(p23;q35) gives rise to NPM1-ALK. The resulting chimeric NPM1-ALK protein homodimerize and the kinase becomes constitutively activated. ALK+ ALCL represent 50 to 60 % of ALCL cases.

  The t(2;5)(p23;q35) translocation is also observed in inflammatory myofibroblastic tumor
- NPM1 is involved in fusions with RARA in a form of acute promyelocytic leukemia (AML-M3). Translocation t(5;17)(q32;q11) gives rise to NPM1-RARA.
- NPM1 is involved in fusions with MLF1 in AML, MDS, CML in blast crisis (BC-CML). Translocation t(3;5)(q25;q34) gives rise to NPM1-MLF1.

NRAS (1p13.2)
Neuroblastoma RAS Viral (V-Ras) Oncogene Homolog

Function
NRAS (Baines et al. 2011) is an oncogene encoding a membrane protein that shuttles between the Golgi apparatus and the plasma membrane. This shuttling is regulated through palmitoylation and depalmitoylation by the ZDHHC9-GOLGA7 complex. The encoded protein, which has intrinsic GTPase activity, is activated to a GTP-bound form by a GTPase activating protein and inactivated to a GDP-bound form by a guanine nucleotide-exchange factor.

Cancer-Related Gene Alterations
- Genetic defects in NRAS are a cause of juvenile myelomonocytic leukemia (JMML), a pediatric myelodysplastic syndrome (MDS) that constitutes approximately 30% of childhood cases of MDS and 2% of leukemia.
- Somatic mutations in NRAS are found in a variety of tumors: skin, bile duct, thyroid, hematopoietic and lymphoid tissue and testis. Most mutation events are substitutions. Somatic mutation hotspots are observed at amino acids 12, 13 and 61.

NTRK3 (15q25)
Neurotrophic Tyrosine Kinase, Receptor, Type 3

Function
NTRK3 encodes a tyrosine-protein kinase receptor for neurotrophin-3. Upon neurotrophin binding, NTRK3 phosphorylates itself and members of the MAPK pathway. Signaling through this kinase leads to neuronal proliferation and differentiation.

Cancer-Related Gene Alterations
- Somatic NTRK3 mutations (mostly substitution missense) have been found in a small (<3%) percentage of lung, skin, stomach and breast tumors. There are no mutation hotspots.
- NTRK3 is involved in fusions with ETV6 in congenital fibrosarcoma and congenital mesoblastic nephroma-cellular variant, which are pediatric tumors of mesoblastic origin. ETV6-NTRK3 gene fusions are the result of a t(12;15)(p13;q25) translocation. This translocation and the resulting fusion gene are also found in secretory breast carcinoma (Weigelt et al. 2010), which is an epithelium-derived breast cancer.

PALB2 (16p12.2)
Partner and Localizer of BRCA2

Function

This gene encodes a protein that may function in tumor suppression (Tischkowitz and Xia 2010). This protein binds to and colocalizes with the breast cancer 2 early onset protein (BRCA2) in nuclear foci and likely permits the stable intranuclear localization and accumulation of BRCA2. It also enables the recombinational repair and checkpoint functions of BRCA2.

Cancer-related Gene Alterations
- Genetic variations in PALB2 are associated with breast cancer susceptibility.
- Defects in PALB2 are the cause of Fanconi Anemia complementation group N (FANCN) (see Fanconi Anemia genes)
- Somatic PALB2 point mutations are rare.

PDGFRA (4q12)
Platelet-Derived Growth Factor Receptor, Alpha Polypeptide

Function

PDGFRA (George 2001) encodes a cell surface tyrosine kinase receptor for members of the platelet-derived growth factor (PDGF) family. These growth factors are mitogens for cells of mesenchymal origin. The identity of the growth factor bound to a receptor monomer determines whether the functional receptor is a homodimer or a heterodimer, composed of both platelet-derived growth factor receptor alpha and beta polypeptides. Activation of PDGFRA kinase activity initiates intracellular signaling through the MAPK, PI3K and PKCγ pathways.

Cancer-related Gene Alterations
- Somatic PDGFRA mutations have been found in tumors of small intestine (about 50% of cases), stomach and soft tissue. Two-thirds of these mutations are

substitution missense, for which a mutation hotspot exists, corresponding to amino acid 842.
- Gastrointestinal stromal tumors (GISTs) are rare neoplasms of mesenchymal origin arising in the gastrointestinal tract. These tumors are characterized by activating mutations of either receptor tyrosine kinase KIT or PDGFRA, which are found in 85% of cases.
- Fusion genes involving PDGFRA and various other genes (FIP1L1, CDK5RAP2, STRN, KIF5B, ETV6, BCR is the cause of diseases accompanied by eosinophilia (see below) :
  - a del(4)(q12q12), leading to IP1L1-PDGFRA, is observed in chronic eosinophilic leukemia (CEL)
  - an ins(9;4)(q33;q12q25), leading to CDK5RAP2-PDGFRA, is observed in CEL
  - a t(2;4)(p22;q12), leading to STRN-PDGFRA, is observed in MPD with eosinophilia
  - a t(4;10)(q12;p11), leading to KIF5B-PDGFRA, is observed in myeloproliferative syndrome (MPS) with hypereosinophilia
  - a t(4;12)(q12;p13), leading to ETV6-PDGFRA, is observed in MPD with hypereosinophilia
  - a t(4;22)(q12;q11.2), leading to BCR-PDGFRA, is observed in MPD and atypical CML

The most investigated of these fusion genes is FIP1L1-PDGFRA.

PHOX2B (4p13)
Paired-Like Homeobox 2b

Function
The DNA-associated protein encoded by this gene (Bourdeaut et al. 2005) is a member of the paired family of homeobox proteins localized to the nucleus. The protein functions as a transcription factor involved in the development of several major noradrenergic neuron populations and the determination of neurotransmitter phenotype. The gene product is linked to enhancement of second messenger-mediated activation of the dopamine beta-hydroylase, c-fos promoters and several enhancers, including cyclic AMP-response element and serum-response element.

Cancer-Related Gene Alterations
- Somatic PHOX2B mutations have been observed almost exclusively in CNS tumors. They are deletions, insertions or substitutions. There are no mutation hotspots.
- Defects in PHOX2B are the cause of susceptibility to neuroblastoma type 2 (NBLST2). NBLST2 is a common neoplasm of early childhood arising from embryonic cells that form the primitive neural crest and give rise to the adrenal medulla and the sympathetic nervous system.

PIK3CA (3q26.3)
Phosphoinositide-3-Kinase, Catalytic, Alpha Polypeptide

Function

PIK3CA (Samuels and Waldman 2010) encodes the p110α protein which is a catalytic subunit of the class I PI 3-kinases (PI3K). Class I PI3K are heterodimeric molecules composed of a catalytic subunit and a regulatory subunit. There are three possible catalytic subunits p110α, β or δ. Class I PI3K are linked to many cellular functions, including cell growth, proliferation, differentiation, motility, survival and intracellular trafficking. PI3K activity may lead in fine to the activation of the Akt/mTOR pathway. PTEN, a tumor suppressor inactivated in many cancers counteracts the action of PI3K.

Cancer-Related Gene Alterations
- PIK3CA is one of the most frequently mutated genes in a wide variety of cancers, for example those affecting colon, breast, urinary tract, endometrium, stomach, cervix, ovary. Defects in PIK3CA are also a cause of seborrheic keratosis, a common benign skin tumor. Most PIK3CA mutations cluster in hotspots within the helical (amino acids 539-546) or the catalytic (kinase, amino acids 1025-1050) domains. Mutations are point substitutions in more than 98% of cases.
- PIK3CA mutations lead to constitutive activation of p110α enzymatic activity and allow growth factor-independent growth. In addition, when expressed in normal cells, these mutations allow anchorage-independent growth, further attesting to their important role in cancer development. PIK3CA gene amplification has also been proposed as a mechanism for oncogene activation in some tumors.

PMS1 (2q31-q33)
PMS1 Postmeiotic Segregation Increased 1 (S. Cerevisiae)

Function

PMS1 (Lynch and de la Chapelle 1999) encodes a protein belonging to the DNA mismatch repair mutL/hexB family. This protein is thought to be involved in the repair of DNA mismatches, and it can form heterodimers with MLH1, a known DNA mismatch repair protein.

Cancer-Related Gene Alterations
- Defects in PMS1 are the cause of hereditary non-polyposis colorectal cancer type 3 (HNPCC3). Mutations in more than one gene locus can be involved alone or in combination in the production of the HNPCC phenotype (also called Lynch syndrome). Most families with clinically recognized HNPCC have mutations in either MLH1 or MSH2 genes.
  HNPCC is an autosomal, dominantly inherited disease associated with marked increase in cancer susceptibility. It is characterized by a familial predisposition to early onset colorectal carcinoma (CRC) and extra-colonic cancers of the gastrointestinal, urological and female reproductive tracts.

HNPCC is reported to be the most common form of inherited colorectal cancer in the Western world, and accounts for 15% of all colon cancers. Cancers in HNPCC originate within benign neoplastic polyps termed adenomas.

PMS2 (7p22.1)
PMS2 Postmeiotic Segregation Increased 2 (S. Cerevisiae)

Function

This gene (Lynch and de la Chapelle 1999) is one of the PMS2 gene family members found in clusters on chromosome 7.

The product of this gene is involved in DNA mismatch repair. It forms a heterodimer with MLH1 and this complex interacts with other complexes bound to mismatched bases.

Cancer-Related Gene Alterations
- Defects in PMS2 are the cause of hereditary non-polyposis colorectal cancer type 4 (HNPCC4). Mutations in more than one gene locus can be involved alone or in combination in the production of the HNPCC phenotype (also called Lynch syndrome).
  Most families with clinically recognized HNPCC have mutations in either MLH1 or MSH2 genes. HNPCC is an autosomal, dominantly inherited disease associated with marked increase in cancer susceptibility. It is characterized by a familial predisposition to early onset colorectal carcinoma (CRC) and extra-colonic cancers of the gastrointestinal, urological and female reproductive tracts. HNPCC is reported to be the most common form of inherited colorectal cancer in the Western world, and accounts for 15% of all colon cancers.
  Cancers in HNPCC originate within benign neoplastic polyps termed adenomas.
- Defects in PMS2 are a cause of mismatch repair cancer syndrome (MMRCS), also known as Turcot syndrome or brain tumor-polyposis syndrome 1 (BTPS1). MMRCS is an autosomal dominant disorder characterized by malignant tumors of the brain associated with multiple colorectal adenomas. Skin features include sebaceous cysts, hyperpigmented and café-au-lait spots.

Polycomb Group (PcG) Proteins

Polycomb group (PcG) proteins (Piunti and Pasini 2011) maintain transcriptional repression of hundreds of genes involved in development, signaling or cancer using chromatin-based epigenetic mechanisms.

Biochemical studies in Drosophila have revealed that PcG proteins associate in at least two classes of protein complexes known as polycomb repressive complexes 1 and 2 (PRC1 and PRC2).

Orthologs have been found in humans. PRC1 proteins include CBX (chromobox homolog) 2, 4, 6, 7 and 8; PHC (polyhomeotic homolog) 1, 2 and 3; BMI1 (B lymphoma Mo-MLV insertion region 1 homolog (mouse)); RING (Ring Finger Protein) 1 and 2; SCMH (sex comb on midleg homolog) 1 and 2; PRC2 proteins include EZH (enhancer of zeste homolog) 1 and 2; EED (embryonic ectoderm development); SUZ12 (suppressor of zeste 12); PHF1 (PHD finger protein 1); other PcG proteins include YY1 (Yin and Yang 1); EPC (enhancer of polycomb homolog) 1 and 2; ASXL (additional sex combs like) 1, 2, and 3.

Among the corresponding genes, ASXL1 (20q11), EZH2 (7q35-q36), and SUZ12 (17q21) are the most frequently mutated. Most SUZ12 alterations are the consequence of translocations leading to SUZ12 gene fusions with JAZF1 and SSH2.

ASXL1 (20q11)
Additional Sex Combs Like 1

Function
ASXL1 plays a role in transcription regulation of differentiation and self-renewal programs. ASXL1 interacts with components of the polycomb complex PRC2, namely EZH2 and SUZ12, two proteins allowing methylation of histone H3 on lysine 27 (H3K27), which serves as an epigenetic mark mediating silencing of gene transcription.

Cancer-Related Gene Alterations
- ASXL1 somatic mutations (insertions, deletions, substitutions) seem to be restricted to hematopoietic and lymphoid tissue tumors. Mutations have been observed in MDS, JMML, CMML, AML, CML, and B-ALL samples. In fact, ASXL1 gene is one of the most frequently mutated genes in malignant myeloid diseases. The most common mutation is an insertion at amino acid 646

EZH2 (7q35-q36)
Enhancer of Zeste Homolog 2

Function
EZH2 is the catalytic subunit of polycomb-repressive complex 2 (PRC2). EZH2 plays a key role in trimethylating Lys27 of histone H3 (H3K27). EZH2 protein may play an important role in the hematopoietic and central nervous systems.

Cancer-Related Gene Alterations
- EZH2 is frequently amplified and/or overexpressed in most solid tumor types.
- Somatic mutations in EZH2 (more than 95% are substitution missense affecting residue Y641 and leading to a gain of methylation function) have been described mostly in hematopoietic and lymphoid tissue tumors.
  These mutations have notably been observed in germinal center B-cell (GCB) diffuse large B-cell lymphomas (DLBCL).and in follicular (FL).

PPP2R1A (19q13.41)
Protein Phosphatase 2, Regulatory Subunit A, A

Function
PPP2R1A (McConechy et al. 2011) encodes the α-isoform of the scaffolding subunit of the serine/threonine protein phosphatase 2A (PP2A) holoenzyme. This putative tumor suppressor complex is involved in growth and survival pathways.

Cancer-Related Gene Alterations
- Somatic mutations, mainly missense, have been found in endometrial cancer, up to 40.8% of samples in high-grade serous endometrial tumors. Mutations were also identified in ovarian tumors at lower frequencies.

PRKAR1A (17q23-q24)
Protein Kinase, Camp-Dependent, Regulatory, Type I, A

Function
cAMP is a signaling molecule important for a variety of cellular functions. cAMP exerts its effects by activating the cAMP-dependent protein kinase "protein kinase A" (PKA), which transduces the signal through phosphorylation of different target proteins. The inactive kinase holoenzyme is a tetramer composed of two regulatory and two catalytic subunits. cAMP causes the dissociation of the inactive holoenzyme into a dimer of regulatory subunits bound to four cAMP and two free monomeric catalytic subunits. Four different regulatory subunits and three catalytic subunits have been identified in humans. PRKAR1A (Bossis and Stratakis 2004) encodes just one of the four regulatory subunits (RIα); however, RIα is the most abundant and widely expressed PKA subunit. Although its other functions are not fully elucidated yet, PRKAR1A may act as a tumor-suppressor gene in Carney complex (CNC) and in sporadic (non-CNC-related) adrenal and thyroid tumors.

Cancer-Related Gene Alterations
- Most germinal mutations in PRKAR1A are null alleles; they are dispersed throughout the coding region of the gene.
- Defects in PRKAR1A are the cause of Carney complex type 1 (CNC1). CNC is a multiple neoplasia syndrome characterized by spotty skin pigmentation, cardiac and other myxomas, endocrine tumors, psammomatous melanotic schwannomas and some other tumors. Half of CNC patients show PRKARIA mutations. PRKARIA is frequently affected by bi-allelic inactivation.
- Defects in PRKAR1A are the cause of primary pigmented nodular adrenocortical disease type 1 (PPNAD1). PPNAD is a rare bilateral adrenal defect causing ACTH-independent Cushing syndrome. Macroscopic appearance of the adrenals is characteristic with small pigmented micronodules observed in the cortex. PPNAD1 is most often diagnosed in patients with Carney complex, but it can also be observed in patients without other manifestations or familial history. Inactivating PRKAR1A germline mutations are frequent in sporadic and isolated cases of PPNAD. Both

alleles are frequently inactivated. The wild-type allele can be inactivated by somatic mutations.
- Defects in PRKAR1A are the cause of intracardiac myxoma. It consists in benign and slowly proliferating lesions that arise from subendocardial pluripotent primitive mesenchymal cells. These lesions can differentiate within myxomas along a variety of lineages including epithelial, hematopoietic, and muscular. Inheritance is autosomal recessive.
- Somatic PRKAR1A mutations have been reported in sporadic adrenocortical tumors. There are no mutation hotspots.
- In papillary thyroid carcinoma, PRKAR1A gene can fuse to the RET protooncogene by translocation (t(10;17)(q11;q24)) and form a thyroid tumor-specific chimeric oncogene RET-PRKAR1A. This fusion leads to the expression of RET in the thyroid cells, where it is normally transcriptionally silent.
- Another translocation, t(17;17)(q21;q24), may fuse PRKAR1A to RARA in AML.

PTCH1 (9q22.32)
Patched 1

Function
The protein encoded by PTCH1 acts as a receptor for "sonic hedgehog", a secreted molecule implicated in the formation of embryonic structures and in tumorigenesis, as well as "indian hedgehog" and "desert hedgehog". PTCH1 associates with the smoothened protein (SMO) to transduce the hedgehog's proteins signal. PTCH1 functions as a tumor suppressor (de Zwaan and Haass 2010). It is thought to have a repressive activity on cell proliferation and could play a role in DNA maintenance, repair and/or replication, since NBCSS syndrome (see below) is a chromosome instability syndrome.

Cancer-Related Gene Alterations
- Germinal PTCH1 mutations lead to protein truncation in nevoid basal cell carcinoma syndrome (NBCCS); mutations types are variable: nucleotide substitutions (missense/nonsense), small deletions, or small insertions mainly, leading to protein truncation; these mutations have been observed in most exons; there is, so far, no mutation hotspot.
- Genetic alterations in PTCH1 are the cause of basal cell nevus syndrome (BCNS) also known as Gorlin syndrome or Gorlin-Goltz syndrome. BCNS is an autosomal dominant disease characterized by nevoid basal cell carcinomas (NBCCS) and developmental abnormalities such as rib and craniofacial alterations, polydactyly, syndactyly, and spina bifida. In addition, the patients suffer from a multitude of tumors like basal cell carcinomas (BCC), fibromas of the ovaries and heart, cysts of the skin, jaws and mesentery, as well as medulloblastomas and meningiomas. PTCH1 is also mutated in squamous cell carcinoma (SCC).
- Somatic mutations and allele loss events have been observed in NBCCS and in sporadic BCC. Mutation and allele loss have also been found in sporadic primitive neuroectodermal tumors (PNETs), sporadic medulloblastomas and in a few cases of esophageal SCC and invasive transitional cell carcinoma of the bladder; mutations

have also been reported in a low frequency of sporadic trichoepitheliomas (tumors often associated with basal cell carcinomas) and in sporadic odontogenic keratocysts. A large majority of these somatic mutations are substitutions. There are no mutation hotspots.

PTEN (10q23)
Phosphatase and Tensin Homolog

Function
Protein product of PTEN (Song et al. 2012) acts as a dual-specificity protein phosphatase, dephosphorylating tyrosine-, serine- and threonine-phosphorylated proteins. It also acts as a lipid phosphatase, an activity that is critical for its tumor suppressor function. By negatively regulating intracellular levels of phosphatidylinositol-3,4,5-trisphosphate in cells, PTEN antagonizes the PI3K-AKT/PKB signaling pathway, thereby modulating cell cycle progression and cell survival.

Cancer-Related Gene Alterations
- Germline PTEN mutations have been documented in Cowden syndrome (CS), Lhermitte-Duclos disease (LDD), Bannayan-Riley-Ruvalcaba syndrome (BRRS) and Proteus syndrome (PS) (see below); these mutations are observed along the various exons of the gene except the 9th (never described) and the 1st (very few reports); a mutational hotspot is observed in exon 5 (amino acids 130-131 and 173) in relation with the catalytic core motif; in the great majority of the cases, inactivating mutations are observed, either by protein truncation, or by missense mutation within the phosphatase domain.
- CS is an autosomal dominant cancer predisposition syndrome associated with elevated risk for tumors of the breast, thyroid and skin. The predominant phenotype for CS is multiple hamartoma syndrome, in many organ systems including the breast (70% of CS patients), thyroid (40-60%), skin, CNS (40%), gastrointestinal tract. Affected individuals are at an increased risk of both breast and thyroid cancers. Trichilemmomas (benign tumors of the hair follicle infundibulum), and mucocutaneous papillomatosis (99%) are hallmarks of CS.
- LDD is characterized by dysplastic gangliocytoma of the cerebellum which often results in cerebellar signs and seizures. LDD and CS seem to be the same entity, and are considered as hamartoma-neoplasia syndromes.
- BRRS has a partial clinical overlap with CS. However, in BRRS, there seems not to be an increased risk of malignancy. BRRS is characterized by the classic triad of macrocephaly, lipomatosis and pigmented macules of the glans penis.
- PS is a hamartomatous disorder characterized by overgrowth of multiple tissues, connective tissue and epidermal naevi, and vascular malformations. Tumors, mostly benign but some malignant, have also been reported in Proteus syndrome, generally presenting by the age of 20 years and including papillary adenocarcinoma of the testis, meningioma, and cystadenoma of the ovaries.
- Somatic PTEN mutations are observed in several tumor types, notably those affecting vulva, endometrium, salivary glands, CNS (glioma), prostate, skin

(malignant melanoma); they lead to a biallelic inactivation of the gene either by homozygous deletion, or by a combination of point mutation (mainly substitution) and a large deletion of the second allele. As with germinal mutations, mutational hot spots correspond to amino acids 130-131 and 173.

- A microdeletion of chromosome 10q23 involving PTEN and BMPR1A is a cause of chromosome 10q23 deletion syndrome. This syndrome shows overlapping features of the following three disorders: BRRS, CS and juvenile polyposis syndrome (JPS).

PTPN11 (12q24.1)
Protein Tyrosine Phosphatase, Non-Receptor Type 11 (Also Named Shp2)

Function
Shp2, the protein encoded by PTPN11 (Grossmann et al. 2010) is a member of the protein tyrosine phosphatase (PTP) family. PTPs are known to be signaling molecules that regulate a variety of cellular processes including cell growth, differentiation, mitotic cycle, and oncogenic transformation. Shp2 is widely expressed in most tissues where it positively controls the activation of the RAS/MAPK cascade induced by several growth factors, and negatively regulates JAK/STAT signaling.

Cancer-Related Gene Alterations
- Germline PTPN11 mutations are involved in Noonan syndrome (NS) type 1, Noonan-like syndrome (NLS) and LEOPARD syndrome.
- NS is a disorder characterized by dysmorphic facial features, short stature, hypertelorism, cardiac anomalies, deafness, motor delay, and a bleeding diathesis. It is a genetically heterogeneous and relatively common syndrome, with an estimated incidence of 1 in 1000-2500 live births. Mutations in PTPN11 account for more than 50% of the cases. Rarely, NS is associated with juvenile myelomonocytic leukemia (JMML). NS1 inheritance is autosomal dominant.
- NLS is an autosomal dominant disorder characterized by Noonan features associated with giant cell lesions of bone and soft tissue.
- LEOPARD syndrome is an autosomal dominant disorder allelic with Noonan syndrome. The acronym LEOPARD stands for lentigines, electrocardiographic conduction abnormalities, ocular hypertelorism, pulmonic stenosis, abnormalities of genitalia, retardation of growth, and deafness.
- Somatic PTPN11 mutations have been documented in a heterogeneous group of hematologic malignancies and pre-leukemic disorders (JMML, AML, ALL, MDS, CML), and rarely in certain solid tumors (melanoma, neuroblastoma, lung adenocarcinoma, colon cancer). A majority of mutations are substitution missense and affect residues residing at or close to the interface between the N-SH2 and PTP domains. There is a mutation hotspot corresponding to amino acid 76. Both germline and somatic mutations promote PTPN11 gain-of-function by destabilizing the catalytically inactive conformation of the protein, and prolong signal flux through the RAS/MAPK pathway in a ligand-dependent manner.

RAD51C (17q25.1)
RAD51 Homolog C (S. Cerevisiae)

Function

The product of RAD51C (Somyajit et al. 2010) is essential for the homologous recombination repair (HRR) pathway of double-stranded DNA breaks arising during DNA replication or induced by DNA-damaging agents.

Cancer-Related Gene Alterations
- Defects in RAD51C are the cause of breast-ovarian cancer familial type 3 (BROVCA3) [for BROVCA1, see BRCA1, for BROVCA2, see BRCA2]. It is a condition associated with familial predisposition to cancer of the breast and ovaries. Characteristic features in affected families are an early age of onset of breast cancer (often before age 50), increased chance of bilateral cancers (cancer that develop in both breasts, or both ovaries, independently), frequent occurrence of breast cancer among men, increased incidence of tumors of other specific organs, such as the prostate.
- Defects in RAD51C are the cause of Fanconi Anemia complementation group O (FANCO) (See Fanconi Anemia pathway).

RB1 (13q14.2)
Retinoblastoma 1

Function

The protein encoded by RB1 (Chinnam and Goodrich 2011) was the first tumor suppressor gene identified. It is a key regulator of entry into cell division. Its active, hypophosphorylated form binds transcription factor E2F1 and represses its transcription activity, leading to cell cycle arrest. RB1 recruits and targets several histone methyltransferases, leading to epigenetic transcriptional repression. RB1 also stabilizes constitutive heterochromatin to maintain the overall chromatin structure. RB1 has many other effects on specific targets depending on the cell type.

Cancer-Related Gene Alterations
- Germinal RB1 mutations are causative for hereditary predisposition to retinoblastoma (RB), which is a congenital malignant tumor that arises from the nuclear layers of the retina. It occurs in about 1:20,000 live births and represents about 2% of childhood malignancies. It is bilateral in about 30% of cases. Although most RB cases appear sporadically, about 20% are transmitted as an autosomal dominant trait with incomplete penetrance. The diagnosis is usually made before the age of 2 years when strabismus or a gray to yellow reflex from pupil ('cat eye') is investigated.
- The spectrum of predisposing RB1 mutations includes large deletions (about 20%), single base substitutions (about 50%) and small length mutations (about 30%); most mutations are associated with almost complete penetrance: some rare alleles show incomplete penetrance and reduced expressivity (low penetrance retinoblastoma)

- Somatic RB1 mutations: in sporadic RB, both RB1 alleles are somatically mutated. Somatic RB1 mutations are found in a variety of tumors affecting eye (about 50% of cases), urinary tract and bladder, endometrium, breast, bone (osteogenic sarcoma), lung, ovary, liver, stomach.
- Deletions, insertions and point mutations are observed. There are no mutational hotspots.

RECQL4 (8q24.3)
RecQ Protein-Like 4

Function

The protein encoded by this gene (Chu and Hickson 2009) is a DNA helicase that belongs to the RecQ helicase family. DNA helicases unwind double-stranded DNA into single-stranded DNAs. RECQL4 suppresses promiscuous genetic recombination and ensures accurate chromosome segregation. This gene is predominantly expressed in thymus and testis.

Cancer-Related Gene Alterations
- Genetic alterations of RECQL4 are a cause of Rothmund-Thomson syndrome (RTS), an autosomal recessive disorder associated with genomic instability, cancer predisposition and premature ageing. RTS is characterized by dermatological features such as atrophy, pigmentation, and telangiectasia and frequently accompanied by juvenile cataract, saddle nose, congenital bone defects, disturbances of hair growth, and hypogonadism.

RET (10q11.2)
Ret Proto-Oncogene

Function

The protein encoded by RET (Phay and Shah 2010) is a tyrosine kinase receptor whose ligands are neurotrophic factors of the glial-cell line derived neurotrophic factor (GDNF) family, including GDNF, neurturin, artemin and persefin. RET plays a crucial role in neural crest development, and it can undergo oncogenic activation *in vivo* and *in vitro* by cytogenetic rearrangement.

Cancer-Related Gene Alterations
- Germline RET mutations cause autosomal dominant inherited multiple endocrine neoplasia type 2 (MEN2A and MEN2B) and familial medullary thyroid carcinoma only (FMTC).
  - MEN2A is the most frequent form of medullary thyroid cancer (MTC). It is an inherited cancer syndrome characterized by MTC, pheochromocytoma (50% of cases) and/or hyperparathyroidism (5 to 20% of cases).
  - MEN2B is an uncommon inherited cancer syndrome characterized by predisposition to MTC and pheochromocytoma which is associated with marfanoid habitus, mucosal neuromas, skeletal and ophtalmic abnormalities, and

ganglioneuromas of the intestine tract. Then the disease progresses rapidly with the development of metastatic MTC and a pheochromocytome in 50% of cases.
- In FMTC, which occurs in 25-30% of MTC cases, MTC is the only clinical manifestation.

  All mutations are missense activating mutations. There are widely dispersed in 7/21 exons of RET with phenotype-genotype relationships: mutations in exon 11 are strongly associated with MEN2A phenotype, mutations in exon 16 or exons 8, 10, 13, 14, 15, with MEN2B and FMTC (rarely MEN2A) phenotypes respectively.

- Germline RET mutations are also associated to the autosomal inherited Hirschprung's disease or colonic aganglionosis (HSCR) which represents 15-20% of HSCR cases. HSCR (1/5000 live births) is a genetic disorder of neural crest development characterized by the absence of intramural ganglion cells in the hindgut, often resulting in intestinal obstruction. Occasionally, MEN2A or FMTC occur in association with HSCR. RET mutations are loss-of-function mutations dispersed throughout the RET coding sequence and include deletions, insertions, frameshift missense and nonsense mutations.

- Somatic RET mutations have been identified in sporadic medullary thyroid carcinoma (MTC), papillary thyroid carcinoma (PTC) and pheochromocytoma.
  - MTC is a common tumor derived from the C cells of the thyroid that typically arises as an irregular, solid or cystic mass from otherwise normal thyroid tissue.
  - PTC is a malignant neoplasm characterized by the formation of numerous, irregular, finger-like projections of fibrous stroma that is covered with a surface layer of neoplastic epithelial cells.
  - Pheochromocytoma is a catecholamine-producing tumor of chromaffin tissue of the adrenal medulla or sympathetic paraganglia. The cardinal symptom, reflecting the increased secretion of epinephrine and norepinephrine, is hypertension, which may be persistent or intermittent.

- Somatic mutations have also been observed in adrenal gland, urinary tract, colorectal cancer and ovarian tumors. A mutational hotspot corresponds to amino acid 918. Substitution missenses are the most frequent mutations.

- Chromosomal aberrations involving RET are found in PTC. Several activating genes rearrange with the RET genomic region coding for the tyrosine kinase domain:
  - Inversion inv(10)(q11.2;q21) generates the RET-CCDC6 oncogene;
  - inversion inv(10)(q11.2;q11.2) generates the RET-NCOA4 oncogene;
  - translocation t(10;14)(q11;q32) with GOLGA5 generates the RET/GOLGA5 oncogene;
  - translocation t(8;10)(p21.3;q11.2) with PCM1 generates the PCM1/RET oncogene;
  - translocation t(6;10)(p21.3;q11.2) with TRIM27 generates the TRIM27-RET oncogene;
  - translocation t(1;10)(p13;q11) with TRIM33 generates the TRIM33-RET oncogene;
  - translocation t(7;10)(q32;q11) with TRIM24 generates the TRIM24-RET oncogene.

- translocation t(1;10)(q21;q11) with NTRK1 generates the NTRK1-RET oncogene ;
- translocation t(10;12)(q11;p13) with ERC1 generates the ERC1-RET oncogene;
- translocation t(10;14)(q11.2;q22.1) with KTN1 generates the KTN1-RET oncogene ;
- translocation t(10;17)(q11;q24) with PRKAR1A generates the PRKAR1A-RET oncogene.

RUNX1 (21q22.3)
Runt-Related Transcription Factor 1

Function

The protein encoded by RUNX1 (Mikhail et al. 2006) is a transcription factor associated with acute myeloid leukemia (AML). It belongs to the Runt-related transcription factor (RUNX) family of genes which are also called core binding factor-α (CBFα). RUNX proteins form a heterodimeric complex with CBFβ which confers increased DNA binding and stability to the complex. RUNX1 is thought to be involved in the development of normal hematopoiesis.

Cancer-Related Gene Alterations
- Somatic RUNX1 mutations (deletion, insertion, point mutations) have been observed in tumors of hematopoietic/lymphoid tissue and CNS. There are no mutational hotspots.
- RUNX1 is frequently mutated in sporadic myeloid and lymphoid leukemia through translocation, point mutation or amplification. It is also responsible for a familial platelet disorder with predisposition to acute myeloid leukemia (FPD-AML).
- Chromosomal alterations involving RUNX1 and leading to fusion genes are well-documented and have been associated with several types of leukemia:
    - ins(8;21)(q22;q22q22) leads to RUNX1-RUNX1T1 in AML
    - ins(21;8)(q22;q13q22) leads to RUNX1-RUNX1T1 in AML
    - ins(21;8)(q22;q21q22) leads to RUNX1-RUNX1T1 in AML
    - t(1;21)(p35;q22) leads to RUNX1-YTHDF2 in AML
    - t(1;21)(p36;q22) leads to RUNX1-PRDM16 in AML, primarily treatment associated (AMLt), MDS
    - t(1;21)(q21;q22) leads to RUNX1-ZNF687 in AML
    - t(2;21)(q11;q22) leads to RUNX1-AFF3 in T-ALL
    - t(3;21)(q26;q22) leads to RUNX1-RPL22P1 in CML, AML, MDS
    - t(3;21)(q26;q22) leads to RUNX1-MDS1 in AMLt, MDS, primarily treatment associated (MDSt)
    - t(3;21)(q26;q22) leads to RUNX1-EVI1 in CML, MDSt, AML, AMLt
    - t(4;21)(q31;q22) leads to RUNX1-SH3D19 in AML
    - t(7;21)(p22;q22) leads to RUNX1-USP42 in AML
    - t(8;21)(q21-q22;q22) leads to RUNX1-RUNX1T1 in AML
    - t(8;21)(q23;q22) leads to ZFPM2-RUNX1 in refractory anemia with excess blasts (RAEB)

- t(8;21)(q24;q22) leads to RUNX1-TRPS1 in T-ALL, AML
- t(11;21)(q13;q22) leads to MACROD1-RUNX in AML, CML, MDS
- t(12;21)(p13;q22) leads to ETV6-RUNX1 in B-ALL
- t(12;21)(q12;q22) leads to RUNX1-CPNE8 in AML
- t(16;21)(q24;q22) leads to RUNX1-CBFA2T3 in MDS, AML, AMLt
- t(X;21)(p22;q22) leads to RUNX1-PRDX4 in AML

- RUNX1 genetic alterations are the cause of familial platelet disorder with associated myeloid malignancy (FPD-AML or FPDMM), which is an autosomal dominant disease characterized by qualitative and quantitative platelet defects, and propensity to develop AML.

SDHA (5p15) and SDHAF2 (11q12.2) and SDHB (1p36.1-p35) and SDHC (1q23.3) and SDHD (11q23) and TMEM127 (2q11.2)
Succinate Dehydrogenase Complex, Subunit A, Flavoprotein Variant and Succinate Dehydrogenase Complex Assembly Factor 2 and Succinate Dehydrogenase Complex, Subunit B, Iron Sulfur (Ip) and Succinate Dehydrogenase Complex, Subunit C, Integral Membrane Protein, 15kda and Succinate Dehydrogenase Complex, Subunit D, Integral Membrane Protein and Transmembrane Protein 127

Function
SDH (Hensen and Bayley 2011) is part of the mitochondrial electron transport chain (complex II, succinate-ubiquinone oxidoreductase) and catalyses the oxidation of succinate to fumarate in the Krebs cycle. Subunits A and B of this complex (SDHA, SDHB) constitute the catalytic core of the enzyme, while SDHC with SDHD anchor the complex to the matrix face of the mitochondrial inner membrane. SDHAF2 is an SDH cofactor that appears to be required for SDHA flavination, stability of the SDH complex, and therefore the function of the SDH enzyme. TMEM127 is a transmembrane protein that control cell proliferation acting as a negative regulator of TOR signaling pathway mediated by mTORC1. It may act as a tumor suppressor. Relationships between SDH and TMEM127 are poorly known.

Cancer-Related Gene Alterations
- Pheochromocytomas (PCC) and paragangliomas (PGL) are rare, usually benign tumors of the sympathetic or parasympathetic paraganglia. Pheochromocytoma is the tumor of the main sympathetic paraganglia, which is the adrenal medulla. The sympathetic paraganglioma secretes catecholamine while the parasympathetic does not. Both of them originate from neural crest cells and share similar mechanisms of tumor development. The same genetic alteration may predispose to the development of sympathetic and parasympathetic paraganglioma. Up to 35% of these tumors may be hereditary; they are associated with germline mutations in genes encoding subunits of the succinate dehydrogenase (SDH) enzyme complex in the context of the familial PGL syndromes, PGL1, 3 and 4 caused by mutations in the SDHD, SDHC and SDHB genes, respectively. Another familial PGL syndrome, PGL2, which is currently exclusively associated with head and neck paragangliomas, is caused by mutations in SDHAF2. Recently mutations were found in the SDHA

subunit in a limited number of patients with PGL and/or PCC. Another gene found to predispose to PGL and/or PCC when mutated is TMEM127.
- The SDHB, SDHC and SDHD gene mutations (but not SDHA) can also be found in patients with PGL and/or PCC and gastrointestinal stromal tumors (GISTs), also known as the Carney-Stratakis syndrome; SDHB mutations, in particular, may also predispose to thyroid and renal cancer, and possibly other tumors.

SETD2 (3p21.31)
SET Domain Containing 2

Function
This protein (Duns et al. 2010) is a histone methyltransferase that is specific for lysine-36 of histone H3, and methylation of this residue is associated with active chromatin. Findings suggest that the histone methyltransferase SETD2 could selectively regulate the transcription of subset genes via cooperation with the transcription factor p53.

Cancer-Related Gene Alterations
- Somatic SETD2 mutations have been observed in a small percentage of kidney (about 5% of cases), breast and skin tumors. They are point mutations (mostly substitutions) or deletions. There are no mutational hotspots.

SF3B1 (2q33.1)
Splicing Factor 3b, Subunit 1, 155kda

Function
The gene encodes a core component of RNA splicing machinery.

Cancer-related Gene Alterations
- Somatic SF3B1 mutations, almost all missense substitutions, have been reported in tumors affecting hematopoietic and lymphoid tissues, notably in cases of myelodysplastic/myeloproliferative neoplasms (Malcovati et al. 2011). In myelodysplasia, there is a significant association of SF3B1 mutations with the presence of ring sideroblasts. There are mutation hotspots corresponding to amino acids 700 (mostly), 666, 662, 625 and 622.

SMAD4 (18q21.1)
SMAD Family Member 4

Function
SMAD4 (Heldin and Moustakas 2012) encodes a member of the Smad family of signal transduction proteins. Smad4 acts as an intracellular mediator of TGF-β family and activin type 1 receptor, to regulate cell growth and differentiation.

Cancer-Related Gene Alterations

- Germline alterations of SMAD4 are a cause of juvenile polyposis syndrome (JPS or JP). JPS is an autosomal dominant gastrointestinal hamartomatous polyposis syndrome in which patients are at risk for developing gastrointestinal cancers. Defects in SMAD4 may also be observed in some patients with juvenile polyposis/hereditary hemorrhagic telangiectasia syndrome (JP/HHT), in which JP and HHT coexist in a single individual. Both JIP and HHT are autosomal dominant disorders, but with distinct and non-overlapping clinical features. HHT is a vascular malformation disorder.
- Somatic mutations in SMAD4 are frequently observed in pancreatic, colorectal, upper aerodigestive tract, thyroid and biliary tract cancers. About one half of these mutations are substitutions. No specific mutation hotspot has been identified. Mutant Smad4 proteins, identified in human carcinomas, were found to be impaired in their ability to regulate gene transcription.

SMO (7q32.1)
Smoothened Homolog (Drosophila)

Function

The hedgehog signaling pathway controls numerous developmental processes. In response to hedgehog, smoothened (Smo), a seven-pass transmembrane protein, orchestrates pathway signaling and controls transcription factor activation. In the absence of hedgehog, the receptor "patched" indirectly inhibits Smo in a catalytic manner.

Cancer-Related Gene Alterations

Somatic SMO mutations have been found in biliary tract (about 10% of cases), skin, large intestine, upper aerodigestive tract and liver tumors. There are no mutational hotspots. Alterations are mostly substitutions.

SOCS1 (16p13.13)
Suppressor of Cytokine Signaling 1

Function

The protein encoded by SOCS1 (Linossi and Nicholson 2012) is a member of the STAT-induced STAT inhibitor (SSI), also known as suppressor of cytokine signaling (SOCS), family. Members of this family are cytokine-inducible negative regulators of cytokine signaling. The SOCS1 protein is rapidly induced following stimulation by several type I and type II cytokines (including IL2, IL3, erythropoietin, CSF2/GM-CSF, and interferon-γ), and it attenuates their signaling by its ability to bind and inhibit all four of the Janus family of intracellular tyrosine kinases (JAKs).

Cancer-Related Gene Alterations
- Somatic SOCS1 mutations have been found in tumors from hematopoietic and lymphoid tissue. Mutations in classical Hodgkin lymphoma and primary mediastinal B-cell lymphoma are frequent. Deletions as well as point mutations are observed. There are no mutational hotspots.

STK11 (19p13.3)
Serine/Threonine Kinase 11

Function
The protein encoded by STK11 is a serine/threonine protein kinase, recently classified as a part of the Ca2+/ calmodulin kinase group of kinases. It phosphorylates and activates members of the adenosine monophosphate-activated protein kinase (AMPK)-related subfamily of protein kinases. In fact, the STK11/AMPK/tuberous sclerosis complex (TSC)/mammalian target of rapamycin (mTOR) complex (mTORC1) cassette is a canonical signaling pathway that integrates information on the metabolic and nutrient status and translates this into regulation of cell growth. Alterations in this pathway are associated with a wide variety of cancers and hereditary hamartoma syndromes, diseases in which hyperactivation of mTORC1 has been described.

STK11 activity is regulated by the pseudokinase STRADα and the scaffolding protein MO25α, resulting in the reorganization of non-polarized cells so they form asymmetrical apical and basal structures.

In addition, STK11 has been implicated in a range of processes including chromatin remodeling, cell cycle arrest (in G1), ras-induced cell transformation, p53-mediated apoptosis and Wnt signaling. STK11 is a tumor suppressor.

Cancer-Related Gene Alterations
- STK11 mutations have been associated with Peutz-Jeghers Syndrome (PJS) (Jansen et al. 2011), which is an autosomal dominant syndrome characterized by a predisposition to benign and malignant tumors of many organ systems. The relative incidence is estimated to vary from 1/29,000 to 1/120,000 births. Features are multiple gastrointestinal tract hamartomous polyps, melanocytic macules on the skin and mouth, and an increased risk for various neoplasms in epithelia tissues. For example it has been estimated that there is a about 84, about 213 and about 520 fold increased risk of developing colon, gastric and small intestinal cancers respectively. PJS patients are also at an increased risk of developing cancers in the breast, lung, ovaries, uterus, cervix and testes.
- A majority (60-70%) of PJS patients show germline mutations in STK11. Patients inherit mutations in one allele, and the remaining allele is later inactivated generally by LOH or sometimes somatic mutation. This biallelic inactivation of STK11 leads to a loss of tumor suppressor activity, thereby promoting tumorigenesis. Genetic locus heterogeneity may exist for this disease. A small percentage of families with no mutations in STK11 have been identified, however no other candidate genes that predispose to PJS have been identified to date.

- Most STK11 germinal mutations identified to date are in the catalytic domain of the protein, indicating that kinase activity is likely essential for its function as a tumor suppressor. Several types of mutations including insertions, deletions, nonsense, missense and splice site alterations have been identified to date. One family has been identified with complete germline deletion of this gene.
- Somatic mutations: many of the polyps that develop in PJS show loss of heterozygosity and sometimes somatic mutations. Somatic mutations (mainly substitutions) rarely occur in sporadic tumors, with the exception of adenocarcinoma of the lung. There are no mutational hotspots, although mutations are slightly more frequent for nucleotides corresponding to amino acids 37, 170 and 354.

SUFU (10q24.32)
Suppressor of Fused Homolog (Drosophila)

Function
The Hedgehog signaling pathway plays an important role in early human development. The pathway is a signaling cascade that plays a role in pattern formation and cellular proliferation during development. The protein encoded by SUFU is a negative regulator in this Hedgehog signaling pathway (Cheng and Yue 2008).

Cancer-Related Gene Alterations
- Genetic alterations in SUFU are a cause of medulloblastoma (MDB), which is a malignant, invasive embryonal tumor of the cerebellum with a preferential manifestation in children. Defects in SUFU play a role in predisposition to desmoplastic MDB. These tumors make up about 20 to 30% of medulloblastomas, have a more nodular architecture than 'classical' medulloblastoma, and may have a better prognosis.

SWI/SNF Complex Components

The SWI/SNF chromatin-remodeling complex (Wilson and Roberts 2011) plays essential roles in a variety of cellular processes including differentiation, proliferation and DNA repair. SWI/SNF is a master regulator of gene expression. In mammalian cells, SWI/SNF has been linked to the expression of: steroid receptors, CD44, CEACAM1, E-cadherin and various integrins, a large number of interferon (IFN)-inducible genes, c-FOS, CSF-1, CRYAB, MIM-1, p21, HSP70, vimentin, cyclindromatosis and cyclin A.

Loss of SWI/SNF subunits has been reported in a number of malignant cell lines and tumors, and a large number of experimental observations suggest that this complex functions as a tumor suppressor.

Genes encoding components of the SWI/SNF complex include ARID1A (AT rich interactive domain 1A (SWI-like)), ARID1B, ARID2, SMARCA2 (SWI/SNF related, matrix associated, actin dependent regulator of chromatin, subfamily a, member 2), SMARCA4, SMARCB1, SMARCC1, SMARCC2, SMARCD1, SMARCD2, SMARCD3, SMARCE1, ACTL6A (Actin-like 6A), ACTL6B, and PBRM1 (Polybromo 1)

ARID1A (1p36.1-p35), ARID1B (6q25.3), ARID2 (12q13.11), PBRM1 (3p21), SMARCA4 (19p13.3) and SMARCB1 (22q11.23) are the most frequently mutated.

Cancer-Related ARID1A Alterations
- Somatic mutations in ARID1A are seen in various tumor types, including ovarian, breast, endometrial, liver, colon, pancreas and gastric cancers. Mutations are substitutions, deletions and insertions and are distributed throughout the gene (no mutation hotspot)
- A mutation study of nine genes: ARID1A, PPP2R1A, PTEN, PIK3CA, KRAS, CTNNB1, TP53, BRAF and PPP2R5C indicated that PTEN, PIK3CA, ARID1A and KRAS mutations were most frequent in "endometrioid-type", while TP53 and PPP2R1A mutations were most frequent in "serous-type" of endometrial carcinomas. Other studies have reported a frequent loss of expression and/or mutation of ARID1A in "endometrioid-type" and "clear cell" carcinomas but only rarely in "serous-type" tumors. Multiple chromatin regulators, including ARID1A, ARID1B, ARID2, MLL and MLL3, appear to be mutated in ~50% of liver tumors. Loss of ARID1A-associated protein expression is a frequent event in clear cell and endometrioid ovarian cancers. In a study of somatic alterations in gastric cancer, frequent mutations in chromatin remodeling genes (ARID1A, MLL3 and MLL) occurred in 47% of gastric cancers. ARID1A mutations were detected in 8% of tumors, which were associated with concurrent PIK3CA mutations and microsatellite instability.

Cancer-Related ARID1B Alterations
- Somatic mutations (mainly substitutions) in ARID1B are seen in various tumor types, including ovarian, breast, liver, pancreas and colon cancers. Mutations are distributed throughout the gene (no mutation hotspot). Multiple chromatin regulators, including ARID1A, ARID1B, ARID2, MLL and MLL3, appear to be mutated in ~50% of liver tumors (Fujimoto et al. 2012). In pancreatic cancer genomes, a study found that genomic deletions, mutations, and rearrangements recurrently targeted genes encoding SWI/SNF complex, including all three putative DNA binding subunits (ARID1A, ARID1B, and PBRM1) and both enzymatic subunits (SMARCA2 and SMARCA4).

Cancer-Related ARID2 Alterations
- Somatic mutations (mainly substitutions) in ARID2 are seen in various tumor types, including ovarian, breast, colon and liver cancers. Mutations are distributed throughout the gene (no mutation hotspot). Inactivating mutations of ARID2 were found in four major subtypes of hepatocellular carcinomas (HCC): HCV-associated HCC, hepatitis B virus (HBV)-associated HCC, alcohol-associated HCC and HCC with no known etiology. Notably, 18.2% of individuals with HCV-associated HCC in the United States and Europe harbored ARID2 inactivation mutations, suggesting that ARID2 is a tumor suppressor gene that is relatively commonly mutated in this tumor subtype.

Cancer-Related PBRM1 Alterations
- PBRM1 encodes the chromatin targeting subunit of the SWI/SNF complex. Somatic PBRM1 mutations (insertions, deletions, substitutions) are particularly frequent in kidney cancer (>30%) and also observed in breast tumors (<5%). No mutation hotspot has been described. It has been reported that PBRM1 is the second major clear cell renal carcinoma gene, after VHL. A study found that BAP1 protein was inactivated in 15% of clear cell renal cell carcinoma (ccRCC). Mutations in BAP1 and PBRM1 were anticorrelated in ccRCC, and combined loss of BAP1 and PBRM1 in a few RCCs was associated with rhabdoid features.

Cancer-Related SMARCA4 Alterations
- SMARCA4 germline mutations have not been reported so far.
- SMARCA4 somatic mutations have been identified in a significant proportion of tumors and cancer cell lines including those from the lung, prostate, breast, pancreas and colon. The type of mutations commonly observed include nonsense, missense and large deletions. No specific mutation hotspot has been described.

Cancer-Related SMARCB1 Alterations
- Various types of SMARCB1 somatic mutations have been described in various tumor types, including soft tissue, CNS, bone and skin tumors. No specific mutation hotspot has been reported.
- Genetic alterations in SMARCB1 are a cause of rhabdoid tumor (RDT). RDT are a highly malignant group of neoplasms that usually occur in early childhood.
- Germline SMARCB1 mutation predisposes to multiple meningiomas and schwannomas with preferential location of cranial meningiomas at the *falx cerebri*. Schwannomas are benign tumors of the peripheral nerve sheath that usually occur singly in otherwise normal individuals. A SMARCB1 exon 2 missense mutation c.143 C > T has been shown to segregate with the presence of meningiomas in five members of a large family with multiple meningiomas and schwannomas.

TBX3 (12q24.1)
T-Box 3

Function
TBX3 (Peres et al. 2010) encodes a member of a phylogenetically conserved family of genes that share a common DNA-binding domain, the T-box. T-box genes encode transcription factors involved in the regulation of developmental processes.

Cancer-Related Gene Alterations
- Somatic TBX3 mutations are observed in tumors affecting breast, ovary and large intestine. They are mainly substitutions. No mutation hotspot has been described.

TET2 (4q24)
Tet (Ten-Eleven-Translocation) Oncogene Family Member 2

Function

The TET proteins (TET1, TET2, TET3) (Abdel-Wahab et al. 2009) are members of the 2-oxoglutarate (2-OG)- and Fe(II)-dependent dioxygenase that are able to convert 5-methylcytosine (5-mC) to 5-hydroxymethylcytosine (hmC). TET2 play an important role in the regulation of myelopoiesis.

Cancer-Related Gene Alterations
- Somatic TET2 mutations are observed in up to 20% of tumors affecting haematopoietic and lymphoid tissues. There are no mutational hotspots. Deletions, insertions, point mutations are found.
- TET2 is frequently mutated in myeloproliferative disorders (MPD). These constitute a heterogeneous group of disorders, also known as myeloproliferative diseases or myeloproliferative neoplasms (MPN), characterized by cellular proliferation of one or more hematologic cell lines in the peripheral blood, distinct from acute leukemia. Included diseases are: essential thrombocythemia, polycythemia vera, primary myelofibrosis (chronic idiopathic myelofibrosis).
- TET2 is frequently mutated in systemic mastocytosis; also known as systemic mast cell disease. It is a clonal disorder of the mast cell and its precursor cells, with features in common with myeloproliferative diseases. The clinical symptoms and signs of systemic mastocytosis are due to accumulation of clonally derived mast cells in different tissues, including bone marrow, skin, the gastrointestinal tract, the liver, and the spleen.
- TET2, followed by ASXL1, RUNX1, TP53 and EZH2, is the most commonly mutated gene in MDS, a heterogeneous group of closely related clonal hematopoietic disorders. All are characterized by a hypercellular or hypocellular bone marrow with impaired morphology and maturation, dysplasia of the myeloid, megakaryocytic and/or erythroid lineages, and peripheral blood cytopenias resulting from ineffective blood cell production. Included diseases are: refractory anemia (RA), refractory anemia with ringed sideroblasts (RARS), refractory anemia with excess blasts (RAEB), refractory cytopenia with multilineage dysplasia and ringed sideroblasts (RCMD-RS). MDS are considered a premalignant condition in a subgroup of patients that often progresses to AML.

TNFAIP3 (6q23-q25)
Tumor Necrosis Factor, Alpha-Induced Protein 3

Function:

TNFAIP3 (Hymowitz and Wertz 2010) is rapidly induced by the tumor necrosis factor (TNF). The protein encoded by this gene has been shown to inhibit NFκB activation as well as TNF-mediated apoptosis. It is critical for limiting inflammatory processes.

Cancer-Related Gene Alterations

- Somatic TNFAIP3 mutations have been identified almost exclusively in hematopoietic and lymphoid tissue tumors (10%-20% of cases). TNFAIP3 is mutated mainly in different subtypes of B-cell lymphomas. It has been identified as tumor suppressor in marginal zone B-cell lymphoma (MZBCL), classical Hodgkin's lymphoma (cHL), diffuse large B-cell lymphoma (DLBCL), and primary mediastinal B-cell lymphoma (PMBL).
- Most TNFAIP3 mutations are nonsense or frameshift and prevent production of full-length TNFAIP3 protein. Deletions are also observed. There are no mutational hotspots.

TP53 (17p13.1)
Tumor Protein P53

Function

TP53 (Goh et al. 2011) encodes p53, a tumor suppressor in many tumor types; it responds to diverse cellular stresses (DNA damage, hypoxia, nucleotide pool depletion, viral infection, oncogene activation) to regulate target genes that induce cell cycle arrest, apoptosis, senescence, DNA repair, or changes in metabolism. The type of effect is depending on the physiological circumstances and on the cell type. P53 is expressed at low level in normal cells and at a high level in a variety of transformed cell lines, where it is believed to contribute to transformation and malignancy.

Mutants of p53 that frequently occur in a number of different human cancers fail to bind the p53 consensus DNA binding site, and hence cause the loss of tumor suppressor activity. Multiple p53 variants due to alternative promoters and multiple alternative splicing have been found. These variants encode distinct isoforms, which can regulate p53 transcriptional activity.

Cancer-Related Gene Alterations

- Germline TP53 alterations may be a cause of Li-Fraumeni (LFS) or Li-Fraumeni-like (LFL) syndromes. LFS is an autosomal dominant familial cancer syndrome that in its classic form is defined as follows: a person diagnosed with sarcoma before age 45 with a first degree relative affected by any tumor before 45 years and another first degree relative with any tumor before 45 years or a sarcoma at any age. LFL is characterized by: a person diagnosed with any childhood cancer, sarcoma, brain tumor, or adrenal cortical tumor before age 45 with a first-degree or second-degree relative diagnosed with a typical LFS cancer (sarcoma, breast cancer, brain cancer, adrenal cortical tumor, or leukemia) at any age and another first-degree or second-degree relative diagnosed with any cancer before age 60. Germline mutation of TP53 is found in about 70% of LFS and 50% of LFL cases. In a few cases of LFS/LFL families free of TP53 mutations, germline mutations in genes connected to the p53 pathway have been found: CHEK2, PTEN, CDKN2A (see these genes).

  In LFS/LFL families affected patients develop a diverse set of malignancies at unusually early ages. Four types of cancers account for 80% of tumors occurring in TP53 germline mutation carriers: breast cancers, soft tissue and bone sarcomas, brain tumors (astrocytomas) and adrenocortical carcinomas. Less frequent tumors include choroid plexus carcinoma or papilloma before the age of 15, rhabdomyosarcoma before the age of 5, leukemia, Wilms tumor, malignant phyllodes tumor, colorectal and gastric cancers.

Of note, germinal mutations of P53 have also been found in families where the criteria for LFS or LFL were not reached.

- Somatic TP53 mutations are observed in about 50% of human cancers and the non-mutated allele is generally lost. The frequency and the type of mutation may vary from one tumor type to another. Indeed, somatic TP53 mutations are frequent in most human cancers, ranging from 3% (in cervical cancer, for instance) to 70% depending on the type, stage and etiology of tumors.

  Most mutations are missense (75%) and others include non-sense (7.5%), deletions, insertions or splicing mutations (17.5%). There are some hotspots for mutations at CpG dinucleotides at codon positions 175, 248, 273 and 282, thus in the specific DNA binding domain of the protein. TP53 gene mutation is a marker of bad prognosis in a number of cancers, such as breast cancer. Specific mutation spectra are observed in lung, liver and skin cancer that are related to specific carcinogen exposure (tobacco smoke, aflatoxin and UV respectively).

- In hematological malignancies, TP53 is genetically altered in less than 5% of acute lymphoblastic leukemia (ALL), but in 60-80% of Hodgkin disease. In skin cancers, TP53 is mutated in 40% of basal cell carcinomas (BCC) and squamous cell carcinomas (SCC) while mutations are infrequent in malignant melanoma. The pattern of TP53 mutation in skin cancer is highly related to UV exposure with a high frequency of CC->TT and C->T transitions and specific hotspots at codons 196 and 278. In breast cancer, the prevalence of mutations is higher in large size, high grade and estrogen receptor negative tumors. It is also higher in BRCA1-related tumors. In lung cancers, most TP53 mutations are linked to exposure to tobacco smoke.

- TP53 alterations are found in Barrett metaplasia a condition in which the normally stratified squamous epithelium of the lower esophagus is replaced by a metaplastic columnar epithelium. The condition develops as a complication in approximately 10% of patients with chronic gastroesophageal reflux disease and predisposes to the development of esophageal adenocarcinoma.

TSC1 (9q34) and TSC2 (16p13.3)
Tuberous Sclerosis 1 and Tuberous Sclerosis 2

Function

Tuberous sclerosis complex (TSC)1 and TSC2 (Orlova and Crino 2010) are tumor suppressors that inhibit cell growth and mutation of either gene causes benign tumors in multiple tissues. The TSC1 and TSC2 gene products form a functional complex that has GTPase-activating protein (GAP) activity toward Ras homolog enriched in brain (Rheb) to inhibit mammalian target of rapamycin complex 1 (mTORC1), which is constitutively activated in TSC mutant tumors.

Cancer-Related Gene Alterations
- Germline TSC1 and/or TSC2 mutations are the cause of tuberous sclerosis complex (TSC). Mutations are inactivating TSC1 by protein truncation. In TSC2, large genomic deletions are observed in <10% of cases; point mutations have been reported; they are widely dispersed, with no cluster; truncating effect is seen in 2/3 of cases. TSC is an autosomal dominant multi-system disorder that affects especially the brain, kidneys, heart, and skin. The molecular basis of TSC is a functional impairment of the hamartin-tuberin complex. TSC is characterized by hamartomas (benign overgrowths predominantly of a cell or tissue type that occurs normally in the organ) and hamartias (developmental abnormalities of tissue combination). Clinical symptoms can range from benign hypopigmented macules of the skin to profound mental retardation with intractable seizures to premature death from a variety of disease-associated causes. Renal cell carcinoma develops occasionally in TSC patients.
- Defects in TSC1 may be a cause of focal cortical dysplasia of Taylor balloon cell type (FCDBC). FCDBC is a subtype of cortical dysplasias linked to chronic intractable epilepsy. Cortical dysplasias display a broad spectrum of structural changes, which appear to result from changes in proliferation, migration, differentiation, and apoptosis of neuronal precursors and neurons during cortical development.
- Defects in TSC2 are a cause of lymphangioleiomyomatosis (LAM). LAM is a progressive and often fatal lung disease characterized by a diffuse proliferation of abnormal smooth muscle cells in the lungs. It affects almost exclusively young women and can occur as an isolated disorder or in association with tuberous sclerosis complex.
- Somatic TSC1 mutations have been observed in urinary tract and bone cancers. No mutation hotspot has been described. Somatic TSC2 mutations have been observed angiomyolipomas and pulmonary LAM cells from women with sporadic LAM

TSHR (14q24-q31)
Thyroid Stimulating Hormone Receptor

Function

TSHR (García-Jiménez and Santisteban 2007) encodes a receptor for thyrothropin (thyroid stimulating hormone or TSH) and plays a major role in controlling thyroid cell metabolism. Its activation stimulates thyroid epithelial cell proliferation, and regulates the expression of differentiation markers such as thyroglobulin, thyroperoxidase and the sodium iodide symporter, necessary for the synthesis of thyroid hormones. TSHR is also activated by other members of the glycoprotein hormone family, including human chorionic gonadotropin, luteinizing hormone and thyrostimulin.

Cancer-Related Gene Alterations
- TSHR mutations may be gain-of-function resulting in constitutional activation of the receptor independently of TSH, or loss-of-function resulting in loss of TSH sensitivity.

- Germline TSHR mutations include missense mutations, nonsense mutations, insertion/deletions, and exon skipping due to alternative splicing. Germinal activating mutations are associated with hereditary or sporadic congenital hyperthyroidism, whereas germinal inactivating mutations are a cause of TSH resistance associated with congenital hypothyroidism and euthyroid hyperthyrotropinemia.
- Somatic TSHR mutations include missense mutations and in-frame deletions. They are observed in about one-third of thyroid tumors (papillary and follicular cancers). There are frequently associated with amino acids 453, 619, 623 and 632. Activating mutations have been identified in hyper-functioning thyroid adenoma and toxic multi-nodular goiter; few cases are associated with thyroid carcinoma. No somatic inactivating mutations have been described so far.

XPA (9q22.3) and ERCC3 (XPB, 2q21) and XPC (3p25) and ERCC2 (XPD, 19q13.3) and DDB2 (XPE, 11p12-p11) and ERCC4 (XPF, 16p13.12) and ERCC5 (XPG, 13q33) and POLH (XPV, 6p21.1)

Xeroderma pigmentosum, complementation group A and Excision repair cross-complementing rodent repair deficiency, complementation group 3 (xeroderma pigmentosum group B complementing) and Xeroderma pigmentosum, complementation group C and Excision repair cross-complementing rodent repair deficiency, complementation group 2 and Damage-specific DNA binding protein 2, 48kDa and Excision repair cross-complementing rodent repair deficiency, complementation group 4 and Excision repair cross-complementing rodent repair deficiency, complementation group 5 and Polymerase (DNA directed), eta

Function

After DNA damage, multiple components are involved in the nucleotide excision repair (NER) pathway, including Xeroderma Pigmentosum (XP) A-G and V (Park and Choi 2006).

The XPA and XPC gene products have been implicated in the first steps of NER, i.e. the recognition of lesions in the DNA. The XPA protein binds to replication protein A (RPA) which enhances the affinity of XPA for damaged DNA and is essential for NER. The XPA protein has been shown to bind to ERCC1 and TFIIH. It is possible that the complex XPA-RPA may tell to the repair machinery which strand contained the damage and therefore should be eliminated. The XPC protein binds to protein HR23B. This XPC-HR23B complex has been implicated in DNA damage recognition. It is very likely that the XPC-HR23B complex is the principal damage recognition complex i.e. essential for the recognition of DNA lesions in the genome. Binding of XPC-HR23B to a DNA lesion causes local unwinding, so that the XPA protein can bind and the whole repair machinery can be loaded onto the damaged site. The XPC-HR23B complex is only required for global genome repair. In case of transcription coupled repair when an RNA polymerase is stalled at a lesion, the DNA is unwound by the transcription complex and XPA can bind independently of XPC-HR23B complex.

ERCC3/XPB gene product has a 3'-5' ATP-dependent helicase activity involved in NER and initiation of basal transcription. It is a subunit of the basal transcription factor TFIIH.

ERCC2/XPD gene product has a 5'-3' ATP-dependent helicase activity involved in NER. It is a subunit of the basal transcription factor TFIIH.

TFIIH fulfills a dual role in transcription initiation and NER and the role of TFIIH in NER might closely mimic its role in the transcription initiation process. In transcription initiation TFIIH is thought to be involved in unwinding of the promoter site to allowing promoter clearance. In the NER process TFIIH causes unwinding of the lesion-containing region that has been localized by XPC-HR23B and XPA-RPA, enabling the accumulation of NER proteins around the damaged site.

DDB2/XPE encodes a protein that is necessary for the repair of ultraviolet light-damaged DNA. This protein is the smaller subunit of a heterodimeric protein complex DDB1/DDB2 that participates in nucleotide excision repair, and this complex mediates the ubiquitylation of histones H3 and H4, which facilitates the cellular response to DNA damage. This subunit appears to be required for DNA binding.

XPF encodes a protein that forms a complex with ERCC1 (XPH, very rarely mutated) and is involved in the 5' incision made during NER.

XPG encodes a protein that is responsible for the 3' incision made during NER.

At the site of a lesion NER proteins create a DNA bubble structure over a length of approximately 25 nucleotides and the XPG protein incises the damaged DNA strand 0-2 nucleotides 3' to the ssDNA-dsDNA junction. In most studies the 3'-incision made by the XPG protein appeared to be performed prior to and independently of the 5'-incision by XPF-ERCC1. The XPG protein is required non-enzymatically for subsequent 5'-incision by the XPF/ERCC1 heterodimer during the NER process.

POLH encodes a DNA polymerase specifically involved in DNA repair. It plays an important role in translesion synthesis, where the normal high fidelity DNA polymerases cannot proceed and DNA synthesis stalls. It has an important function in the repair of UV-induced pyrimidine dimers.

Cancer-Related Gene Alterations

- XPA, ERCC3 (XPB), XPC, ERCC2 (XPD), DDB2 (XPE), ERCC4 (XPF), ERCC5 (XPG) and POLH (XPV) are involved in the development of Xeroderma Pigmentosum (XP). XP patients are characterized by a progressive degeneration of sun-exposed areas of the skin and eyes. Some patients also manifest with progressive neurologic degeneration. Individuals with XP who are younger than age 20 years have a greater than 1000-fold increased risk of cancer at UV-exposed sites including the skin and eyes. The median age of onset of non-melanoma skin cancer is before age ten years. Among the eight alleles which may play a role in manifestations of XP, seven are involved in processes of nucleic excision repair (NER): XPA, ERCC3 (XPB), XPC, ERCC2 (XPD), DDB2 (XPE), ERCC4 (XPF), ERCC5 (XPG); an additional class of patients referred to as XP variants (XPV) result from deficiencies in POLH, a gene involved in semi-conservative replication of previously damaged sites in DNA.
- About 50% of XP are associated to mutations in XPA or XPC (see below). Compared to XPB, XPD is altered in about 15% of XP. This is probably because, contrarily to the XPB helicase, the helicase activity of XPD is indispensable for NER but not for transcription initiation. So, there is much more XPD patients.

XPA	25%
ERCC3 (XPB)	Rare
XPC	25%
ERCC2 (XPD)	15%
DDB2	Rare
ERCC4 (XPF)	6%
ERCC5 (XPG)	6%
POLH (XPV)	21%

- Somatic mutations of XP genes are rarely observed.
- Three disorders, not directly linked to cancer, may be genetically related to XP: trichothiodystrophy (TTD), Cockayne syndrome (CS) and cerebrooculofacioskeletal syndrome (COFS).

WRN (8p12)
Werner Syndrome, Recq Helicase-Like

Function
This gene encodes a DNA helicase (Chu and Hickson 2009). The protein possesses an intrinsic 3' to 5' DNA helicase activity, and is also a 3' to 5' exonuclease. It functionally interacts with DNA polymerase δ (POLD1) and replication protein A (RPA) complex, which are required for DNA replication and DNA repair, with Ku70/80 heterodimer which is involved in double strand DNA break repair by non-homologous DNA end joining, and with p53.

Cancer-Related Gene Alterations
- WRN mutations are a cause of Werner syndrome (WS). WS is a rare autosomal recessive progeroid syndrome characterized by the premature onset of multiple age-related disorders, including atherosclerosis, cancer, non-insulin-dependent diabetes mellitus, ocular cataracts and osteoporosis. The major cause of death, at a median age of 47, is myocardial infarction. To date, all known WRN mutations produces prematurely terminated proteins.
- Germinal mutations in WRN are located over the entire gene and include stop codons, insertions/deletions and exon deletions: not a single missense mutation has been identified so far.
- Somatic mutations in WRN have been associated with colon cancer. These mutations are substitutions.

WT1 (11p13)
Wilms Tumor 1

Function
WT1 (Huff 2011) encodes a transcription factor that plays an important role in cellular development and cell survival. It has an essential role in the normal development of the

urogenital system. It has a tumor suppressor as well as an oncogenic role in tumor formation. It is highly expressed in the developing kidney.

Cancer-Related Gene Alterations
- Various types of germline mutations have been observed in WT1, mostly affecting zinc fingers in exons 7-10.
- WT1 alterations may be the cause of Wilms tumor (WT), WAGR syndrome, Frasier syndrome (FS), Denys-Drash syndrome (DDS), and desmoplastic small round cell tumor (DSRCT).
- WT is an embryonal malignancy of the kidney that affects approximately 1 in 10,000 infants and young children. It occurs both in sporadic and hereditary forms.
- WAGR syndrome is a rare genetic syndrome in which affected children are predisposed to develop Wilms tumor, gonadoblastoma, aniridia, and mental retardation. WAGR syndrome is caused by a mutation at chromosomal region 11p13. Specifically, several genes in this area are deleted, including the PAX6 ocular development gene and the Wilms tumor gene (WT1).
- FS is characterized by a slowly progressing nephropathy leading to renal failure in adolescence or early adulthood, male pseudohermaphroditism, and no Wilms tumor. There is phenotypic overlap with Denys-Drash syndrome. Inheritance is autosomal dominant.
- DDS is a typical nephropathy characterized by diffuse mesangial sclerosis, genital abnormalities, and/or Wilms tumor. There is phenotypic overlap with WAGR syndrome and Frasier syndrome. Inheritance is autosomal dominant, but most cases are sporadic.
- In DSRCT, a t(11;22)(p13;q12) translocation leads to an in frame fusion of EWSR1 exons 1-7 and WT1 exons 8-10, and to an abnormal EWSR1-WT1 protein.
- Somatic alterations: biallelic WT1 inactivation has been found in Wilms tumors (<15%) and in some mesotheliomas and granulosa cell tumors. Somatic WT1 alterations have been observed in kidney and in hematopoietic and lymphoid tissue (in myelodysplastic syndrome in progression and in acute leukemia). These alterations are insertions or substitutions and are frequent in a gene region corresponding to amino acids 300-316.

References

Abdel-Wahab O, Mullally A, Hedvat C, Garcia-Manero G, Patel J, Wadleigh M, Malinge S, Yao J, Kilpivaara O, Bhat R, et al. Genetic characterization of TET1, TET2, and TET3 alterations in myeloid malignancies. *Blood.* 2009 Jul 2;114(1):144-7.

Antoni L, Sodha N, Collins I, Garrett MD. CHK2 kinase: cancer susceptibility and cancer therapy - two sides of the same coin? *Nat Rev Cancer.* 2007 Dec;7(12):925-36.

Armendariz AD, Krauss RM. Hepatic nuclear factor 1-alpha: inflammation, genetics, and atherosclerosis. *Curr Opin Lipidol.* 2009 Apr;20(2):106-11.

Baines AT, Xu D, Der CJ. Inhibition of Ras for cancer treatment: the search continues. *Future Med Chem.* 2011 Oct;3(14):1787-808.

Balogh K, Patócs A, Hunyady L, Rácz K. Menin dynamics and functional insight: take your partners. *Mol Cell Endocrinol.* 2010 Sep 15;326(1-2):80-4.

Battaglia S, Maguire O, Campbell MJ. Transcription factor co-repressors in cancer biology: roles and targeting. *Int J Cancer.* 2010 Jun 1;126(11):2511-9.

Bellam N, Pasche B.Tgf-beta signaling alterations and colon cancer. *Cancer Treat Res.* 2010;155:85-103.

Borodovsky A, Seltzer MJ, Riggins GJ. Altered cancer cell metabolism in gliomas with mutant IDH1 or IDH2. *Curr Opin Oncol.* 2012 Jan;24(1):83-9.

Bossis I, Stratakis CA. Minireview: PRKAR1A: normal and abnormal functions. *Endocrinology.* 2004 Dec;145(12):5452-8.

Bourdeaut F, Trochet D, Janoueix-Lerosey I, Ribeiro A, Deville A, Coz C, Michiels JF, Lyonnet S, Amiel J, Delattre O. Germline mutations of the paired-like homeobox 2B (PHOX2B) gene in neuroblastoma. *Cancer Lett.* 2005 Oct 18;228(1-2):51-8.

Cantor SB, Guillemette S. Hereditary breast cancer and the BRCA1-associated FANCJ/BACH1/BRIP1. *Future Oncol.* 2011 Feb;7(2):253-61.

Carbone M, Korb Ferris L, Baumann F, Napolitano A, Lum CA, Flores EG, Gaudino G, Powers A, Bryant-Greenwood P, Krausz T, Hyjek E, Tate R, Friedberg J, Weigel T, Pass HI, Yang H. BAP1 cancer syndrome: malignant mesothelioma, uveal and cutaneous melanoma, and MBAITs. *J Transl Med.* 2012 Aug 30;10(1):179.

Chédin F. The DNMT3 family of mammalian de novo DNA methyltransferases. *Prog Mol Biol Transl Sci.* 2011;101:255-85.

Cheng SY, Yue S. Role and regulation of human tumor suppressor SUFU in Hedgehog signaling. *Adv Cancer Res.* 2008;101:29-43.

Chinnam M, Goodrich DW. RB1, development, and cancer. *Curr Top Dev Biol.* 2011;94:129-69.

Chou FS, Mulloy JC. The thrombopoietin/MPL pathway in hematopoiesis and leukemogenesis. *J Cell Biochem.* 2011 Jun;112(6):1491-8.

Chou J, Provot S, Werb Z. GATA3 in development and cancer differentiation: cells GATA have it! *J Cell Physiol.* 2010 Jan;222(1):42-9.

Chu WK, Hickson ID. RecQ helicases: multifunctional genome caretakers. *Nat Rev Cancer.* 2009 Sep;9(9):644-54.

Clevers H, Nusse R. Wnt/β-catenin signaling and disease. *Cell.* 2012 Jun 8;149(6):1192-205.

Crispino JD. GATA1 in normal and malignant hematopoiesis. *Semin Cell Dev Biol.* 2005 Feb;16(1):137-47.

Cuenda A. Mitogen-activated protein kinase kinase 4 (MKK4). *Int J Biochem Cell Biol.* 2000 Jun;32(6):581-7.

Dang CV. MYC on the path to cancer. *Cell.* 2012 Mar 30;149(1):22-35.

De Braekeleer E, Douet-Guilbert N, Rowe D, Bown N, Morel F, Berthou C, Férec C, De Braekeleer M. ABL1 fusion genes in hematological malignancies: a review. *Eur J Haematol.* 2011 May;86(5):361-71.

Derheimer FA, Kastan MB. Multiple roles of ATM in monitoring and maintaining DNA integrity. *FEBS Lett.* 2010 Sep 10;584(17):3675-81.

de Zwaan SE, Haass NK. Genetics of basal cell carcinoma. *Australas J Dermatol.* 2010 May;51(2):81-92.

Duns G, van den Berg E, van Duivenbode I, Osinga J, Hollema H, Hofstra RM, Kok K. Histone methyltransferase gene SETD2 is a novel tumor suppressor gene in clear cell renal cell carcinoma. *Cancer Res.* 2010 Jun 1;70(11):4287-91.

Falini B, Martelli MP, Bolli N, Sportoletti P, Liso A, Tiacci E, Haferlach T. Acute myeloid leukemia with mutated nucleophosmin (NPM1): is it a distinct entity? *Blood.* 2011 Jan 27;117(4):1109-20.

Fletcher JA, Rubin BP. KIT mutations in GIST. *Curr Opin Genet Dev.* 2007 Feb;17(1):3-7.

Fulda S. Caspase-8 in cancer biology and therapy. *Cancer Lett.* 2009 Aug 28;281(2):128-33.

García-Jiménez C, Santisteban P. TSH signalling and cancer. *Arq Bras Endocrinol Metabol.* 2007 Jul;51(5):654-71.

George D. Platelet-derived growth factor receptors: a therapeutic target in solid tumors. *Semin Oncol.* 2001 Oct;28(5 Suppl 17):27-33.

Goh AM, Coffill CR, Lane DP. The role of mutant p53 in human cancer. *J Pathol.* 2011 Jan;223(2):116-26.

Grossmann KS, Rosário M, Birchmeier C, Birchmeier W. The tyrosine phosphatase Shp2 in development and cancer. *Adv Cancer Res.* 2010;106:53-89.

Heldin CH, Moustakas A. Role of Smads in TGFβ signaling. *Cell Tissue Res.* 2012 Jan;347(1):21-36.

Hensen EF, Bayley JP. Recent advances in the genetics of SDH-related paraganglioma and pheochromocytoma. *Fam Cancer.* 2011 Jun;10(2):355-63.

Heron-Milhavet L, Khouya N, Fernandez A, Lamb NJ. Akt1 and Akt2: differentiating the aktion. *Histol Histopathol.* 2011 May;26(5):651-62.

Huff V. Wilms' tumours: about tumour suppressor genes, an oncogene and a chameleon gene. *Nat Rev Cancer.* 2011 Feb;11(2):111-21.

Hymowitz SG, Wertz IE. A20: from ubiquitin editing to tumour suppression. *Nat Rev Cancer.* 2010 May;10(5):332-41.

Jansen M, Langeveld D, De Leng WW, Milne AN, Giardiello FM, Offerhaus GJ. LKB1 as the ghostwriter of crypt history. *Fam Cancer.* 2011 Sep;10(3):437-46.

Kennedy RD, D'Andrea AD. The Fanconi Anemia/BRCA pathway: new faces in the crowd. *Genes Dev.* 2005 Dec 15;19(24):2925-40.

Kim MK, Min DJ, Rabin M, Licht JD. Functional characterization of Wilms tumor-suppressor WTX and tumor-associated mutants. *Oncogene.* 2011 Feb 17;30(7):832-42.

Kim WY, Sharpless NE. The regulation of INK4/ARF in cancer and aging. *Cell.* 2006 Oct 20;127(2):265-75.

Knipscheer P, Räschle M, Smogorzewska A, Enoiu M, Ho TV, Schärer OD, Elledge SJ, Walter JC. The Fanconi anemia pathway promotes replication-dependent DNA interstrand cross-link repair. *Science.* 2009 Dec 18;326(5960):1698-701.

Knowles MA. Role of FGFR3 in urothelial cell carcinoma: biomarker and potential therapeutic target. *World J Urol.* 2007 Dec;25(6):581-93.

Langdon WY. FLT3 signaling and the development of inhibitors that target FLT3 kinase activity. *Crit Rev Oncog.* 2012;17(2):199-209.

Lee J, Kim SS. The function of p27 KIP1 during tumor development. *Exp Mol Med.* 2009 Nov 30;41(11):765-71.

Linossi EM, Nicholson SE. The SOCS box-adapting proteins for ubiquitination and proteasomal degradation. *IUBMB Life.* 2012 Apr;64(4):316-23.

Lynch HT, de la Chapelle A. Genetic susceptibility to non-polyposis colorectal cancer. *J Med Genet.* 1999 Nov;36(11):801-18.

Malcovati L, Papaemmanuil E, Bowen DT, Boultwood J, Della Porta MG, Pascutto C, Travaglino E, Groves MJ, Godfrey AL, Ambaglio I, et al. Clinical significance of SF3B1 mutations in myelodysplastic syndromes and myelodysplastic/myeloproliferative neoplasms. *Blood.* 2011 Dec 8;118(24):6239-46.

Marti TM, Kunz C, Fleck O. DNA mismatch repair and mutation avoidance pathways. *J Cell Physiol.* 2002 Apr;191(1):28-41.

Massoumi R. CYLD: a deubiquitination enzyme with multiple roles in cancer. *Future Oncol.* 2011 Feb;7(2):285-97.

McConechy MK, Anglesio MS, Kalloger SE, Yang W, Senz J, Chow C, Heravi-Moussavi A, Morin GB, Mes-Masson AM; Australian Ovarian Cancer Study Group, et al. Subtype-specific mutation of PPP2R1A in endometrial and ovarian carcinomas. *J Pathol.* 2011 Apr;223(5):567-73.

Mikhail FM, Sinha KK, Saunthararajah Y, Nucifora G. Normal and transforming functions of RUNX1: a perspective. *J Cell Physiol.* 2006 Jun;207(3):582-93.

Minde DP, Anvarian Z, Rüdiger SG, Maurice MM. Messing up disorder: how do missense mutations in the tumor suppressor protein APC lead to cancer? *Mol Cancer.* 2011 Aug 22;10:101.

Moran CJ, Joyce M, McAnena OJ. CDH1 associated gastric cancer: a report of a family and review of the literature. *Eur J Surg Oncol.* 2005 Apr;31(3):259-64.

Narla G, Friedman SL, Martignetti JA. Krüppel cripples prostate cancer: KLF6 progress and prospects. *Am J Pathol.* 2003 Apr;162(4):1047-52.

Ogawa S, Shih LY, Suzuki T, Otsu M, Nakauchi H, Koeffler HP, Sanada M. Deregulated intracellular signaling by mutated c-CBL in myeloid neoplasms. *Clin Cancer Res.* 2010 Aug 1;16(15):3825-31.

Oh ST, Gotlib J. JAK2 V617F and beyond: role of genetics and aberrant signaling in the pathogenesis of myeloproliferative neoplasms. *Expert Rev Hematol.* 2010 Jun;3(3):323-37.

Orlova KA, Crino PB. The tuberous sclerosis complex. *Ann N Y Acad Sci.* 2010 Jan;1184:87-105.

Palomero T, Ferrando A. Oncogenic NOTCH1 control of MYC and PI3K: challenges and opportunities for anti-NOTCH1 therapy in T-cell acute lymphoblastic leukemias and lymphomas. *Clin Cancer Res.* 2008 Sep 1;14(17):5314-7.

Park CJ, Choi BS. The protein shuffle. Sequential interactions among components of the human nucleotide excision repair pathway. *FEBS J.* 2006 Apr;273(8):1600-8.

Paz-Priel I, Friedman A. C/EBPα dysregulation in AML and ALL. *Crit Rev Oncog.* 2011;16(1-2):93-102.

Peña-Llopis S, Vega-Rubín-de-Celis S, Liao A, Leng N, Pavía-Jiménez A, Wang S, Yamasaki T, Zhrebker L, Sivanand S, Spence P, et al. BAP1 loss defines a new class of renal cell carcinoma. *Nat Genet.* 2012 Jun 10;44(7):751-9.

Peres J, Davis E, Mowla S, Bennett DC, Li JA, Wansleben S, Prince S. The Highly Homologous T-Box Transcription Factors, TBX2 and TBX3, Have Distinct Roles in the Oncogenic Process. *Genes Cancer.* 2010 Mar;1(3):272-82.

Phay JE, Shah MH. Targeting RET receptor tyrosine kinase activation in cancer. *Clin Cancer Res.* 2010 Dec 15;16(24):5936-41.

Piunti A, Pasini D. Epigenetic factors in cancer development: polycomb group proteins. *Future Oncol.* 2011 Jan;7(1):57-75.

Röring M, Brummer T. Aberrant B-Raf signaling in human cancer -- 10 years from bench to bedside. *Crit Rev Oncog.* 2012;17(1):97-121.

Roy R, Chun J, Powell SN. BRCA1 and BRCA2: different roles in a common pathway of genome protection. *Nat Rev Cancer.* 2011 Dec 23;12(1):68-78.

Samuels Y, Waldman T. Oncogenic mutations of PIK3CA in human cancers. Curr *Top Microbiol Immunol.* 2010;347:21-41.

Seshacharyulu P, Ponnusamy MP, Haridas D, Jain M, Ganti AK, Batra SK. Targeting the EGFR signaling pathway in cancer therapy. *Expert Opin Ther Targets.* 2012 Jan;16(1):15-31.

Sisley K, Doherty R, Cross NA. What hope for the future? GNAQ and uveal melanoma. *Br J Ophthalmol.* 2011 May;95(5):620-3.

Sjöblom T, Jones S, Wood LD, Parsons DW, Lin J, Barber TD, Mandelker D, Leary RJ, Ptak J, Silliman N, et al. The consensus coding sequences of human breast and colorectal cancers. *Science.* 2006 Oct 13;314(5797):268-74.

Somyajit K, Subramanya S, Nagaraju G. RAD51C: a novel cancer susceptibility gene is linked to Fanconi anemia and breast cancer. *Carcinogenesis.* 2010 Dec;31(12):2031-8.

Song MS, Salmena L, Pandolfi PP. The functions and regulation of the PTEN tumour suppressor. *Nat Rev Mol Cell Biol.* 2012 Apr 4;13(5):283-96.

Stephens PJ, Tarpey PS, Davies H, Van Loo P, Greenman C, Wedge DC, Nik-Zainal S, Martin S, Varela I, Bignell GR, Yates LR, Papaemmanuil E, et al. The landscape of cancer genes and mutational processes in breast cancer. Nature. 2012 May 16;486(7403):400-4.

Tirado CA, Valdez F, Klesse L, Karandikar NJ, Uddin N, Arbini A, Fustino N, Collins R, Patel S, Smart RL, et al. Acute myeloid leukemia with inv(16) with CBFB-MYH11, 3'CBFB deletion, variant t(9;22) with BCR-ABL1, and del(7)(q22q32) in a pediatric patient: case report and literature review. *Cancer Genet Cytogenet.* 2010 Jul 1;200(1):54-9.

Tischkowitz M, Xia B. PALB2/FANCN: recombining cancer and Fanconi anemia. *Cancer Res.* 2010 Oct 1;70(19):7353-9.

Toro JR, Wei MH, Glenn GM, Weinreich M, Toure O, Vocke C, Turner M, Choyke P, Merino MJ, Pinto PA, *et al.* BHD mutations, clinical and molecular genetic investigations of Birt-Hogg-Dubé syndrome: a new series of 50 families and a review of published reports. *J Med Genet.* 2008 Jun;45(6):321-31.

Verdin H, De Baere E. FOXL2 impairment in human disease. *Horm Res Paediatr.* 2012;77(1):2-11.

Vogelstein B, Kinzler KW. Cancer genes and the pathways they control. *Nat Med.* 2004 Aug;10(8):789-99.

Wan X, Choh Y, Kim SY, Dolan JG, Ngo VN, Burkett S, Khan J, Staudt LM, Helman LJ. Identification of the FoxM1/Bub1b signaling pathway as a required component for growth and survival of rhabdomyosarcoma. *Cancer Res.* 2012 Sep 20. [Epub ahead of print]

Wang W. Emergence of a DNA-damage response network consisting of Fanconi anaemia and BRCA proteins. *Nat Rev Genet.* 2007 Oct;8(10):735-48.

Weigelt B, Geyer FC, Reis-Filho JS. Histological types of breast cancer: how special are they? *Mol Oncol.* 2010 Jun;4(3):192-208.

Weinstein LS, Liu J, Sakamoto A, Xie T, Chen M. Minireview: GNAS: normal and abnormal functions. *Endocrinology.* 2004 Dec;145(12):5459-64.

Welcker M, Clurman BE. FBW7 ubiquitin ligase: a tumour suppressor at the crossroads of cell division, growth and differentiation. *Nat Rev Cancer.* 2008 Feb;8(2):83-93.

Wilson BG, Roberts CW. SWI/SNF nucleosome remodellers and cancer. *Nat Rev Cancer.* 2011 Jun 9;11(7):481-92.

Wuyts W, Van Hul W. Molecular basis of multiple exostoses: mutations in the EXT1 and EXT2 genes. *Hum Mutat.* 2000;15(3):220-7.

Yauch RL, Settleman J. Recent advances in pathway-targeted cancer drug therapies emerging from cancer genome analysis. *Curr Opin Genet Dev.* 2012 Feb;22(1):45-9.

Yogev O, Yogev O, Singer E, Shaulian E, Goldberg M, Fox TD, Pines O. Fumarase: a mitochondrial metabolic enzyme and a cytosolic/nuclear component of the DNA damage response. *PLoS Biol.* 2010 Mar 9;8(3):e1000328.

Yohay KH. The genetic and molecular pathogenesis of NF1 and NF2. *Semin Pediatr Neurol.* 2006 Mar;13(1):21-6.

Zorcolo L, Fantola G, Balestrino L, Restivo A, Vivanet C, Spina F, Cabras F, Ambu R, Casula G. MUTYH-associated colon disease: adenomatous polyposis is only one of the possible phenotypes. A family report and literature review. *Tumori.* 2011 Sep-Oct;97(5):676-80.

Chapter 2

Gene Fusions in Cancer

Abstract

Cancer is frequently associated to chromosomal rearrangements (deletions, insertions, inversions, translocations…), of which some may lead to fusions between different genes. Various hybrids have been shown to play a causative role in cancer development or progression. Most of these hybrids have been identified in hematological cancers. However, an increasing number of rearrangements events are now described in tumors of mesenchymal or epithelial origin.

Introduction

Chromosomal rearrangements (deletions, insertions, inversions, translocations…) that lead to gene fusions are among the most common somatic aberrations in cancers. Hundreds of recurrent fusion genes have been discovered in tumors. Most of these hybrids have been identified in hematological cancers. However, an increasing number of rearrangements events are described in tumors of mesenchymal or epithelial origin. Gene fusions are of interest not only because they may often be used as ideal markers which are specific for disease entities or for tumor subtypes. Another reason is that hybrid proteins resulting from chimeric genes may play a key role in malignant transformation and cancer development, and thus constitute potential targets for specific therapies.

Fused Genes

The "Philadelphia chromosome", described in 1960 in CML (Nowell and Hungerford 1960), was the first example of a consistent aberrant autosomal chromosome in a human cancer. It was later demonstrated that this Philadelphia chromosome was a reciprocal chromosomal translocation involving chromosome 9 and chromosome 22, t(9;22)(q34;q11), and that this translocation led to the fusion of the BCR and ABL1 genes, giving rise to an oncogenic fusion protein exhibiting a constitutively active tyrosine kinase activity. BCR-

ABL1, observed in 100% of CML cases and in B-cell ALL, has allowed the development of efficient compounds that selectively inhibit tyrosine kinase (imatinib, nilotinib, dasatinib, bosutinib...) (Kantarjian et al. 2011). This illustrates how specific alterations, once identified in a specific type of cancer, may be the basis for the introduction of new specific targeted therapies.

Since the 1960s, many recurrent gene fusions have been characterized in human cancers (for a review, see (Mitelman et al. 2007)). Different tumor types may be associated to different fusion events, involving specific genes. For instance, MLL, EWSR1, and RET may have many different fusion partners contributing to leukemia, sarcoma, or carcinoma, respectively (Rabbitts 1994). In patients with AML and ALL, MLL has been found to be fused to more than 60 different partner genes. MLL is believed to regulate homeotic genes that are transcriptional activators that are transcriptionally regulated gene families (Bernt and Armstrong 2011). In leukemia, ABL1 may be fused not only to BCR, but also to ETV6, ZMIZ1, EML1, NUP214, SFPQ and RCSD1 (De Braekeleer et al. 2011). On the other hand, some gene fusions may be found in various tumor types: this is notably exemplified by ETV6-NTRK3 (resulting from t(12;15)(p13;q25)), observed in congenital fibrosarcoma, congenital mesoblastic nephroma, secretory breast carcinoma, and AML (Lannon and Sorensen 2005), or by TPM3-ALK (from t(1;2)(q25;p23)), found in IMT, ALCL and, more recently, in renal cell carcinoma (Sugawara et al. 2012).

Some gene fusions are more frequent than others. For instance, in AML, RUNX1-RUNX1T1, resulting from t(8;21)(q22;q22) and PML-RARA (from t(15:17)(q22;q21)) are observed in about 4,2% of cases (Mrózek and Bloomfield 2008), while the frequency of RBM15-MKL1 (t(1;22)(p13;q13)) or MYST3-CREBBP (t(8;16)(p11;p13)) is only 0,1%.

Various oncogenes may be activated as a consequence of chromosomal translocations resulting in a new transcriptional environment. This is notably observed in hematopoietic neoplasias where TCR (encoding the T cell receptor) or IG (encoding immunoglobulins) genes are involved (for example, see (Aifantis et al. 2008)).

Initially, most gene fusion events were observed in hematological cancers, raising some doubts about their commonness in solid tumors. However, throughout the 1990s and 2000s, gene fusions were described in a growing number of mesenchymal tumors. The observation of gene fusions in various epithelial tumors is even more recent. Indeed, in 2004, hematological malignancies, which constitute less than 10% of all human cancers, accounted for about 80% of all known recurrent balanced chromosomal aberrations. In contrast, malignant epithelial tumors which cause 80% of human cancer-related deaths, constituted only 10% of all known recurrent balanced chromosomal aberrations (Kumar-Sinha et al. 2006). The first example of "epithelial" gene fusion, RET-CCDC6, was found in papillary thyroid carcinoma, the most prevalent form of thyroid cancer, in the early 1990s (Pierotti et al. 1992). It has been shown since that the tyrosine kinase receptor RET is a major partner in fusions observed in thyroid cancer, participating to at least 10 different events. Another frequent partner, NTRK3, is also a tyrosine kinase receptor. It appears that, when fused to various other partners, both proteins, which are normally membrane-bound, lose their N-terminal signal peptide and become cytoplasmic. This leads to a constitutive tyrosine-kinase activity. Since the initial findings in thyroid cancers, other gene fusions have been discovered in carcinomas (Mitelman et al. 2007). In salivary glands, they often involve PLAG1 and HMGA2, which encode transcription factors involved in growth factor signaling and cell cycle regulation. However, in mucoepidermoid carcinoma, the most common malignant salivary gland tumor, gene fusions frequently involve MAML2, creating a fusion product that disrupts a Notch signaling pathway. In renal cancers, many fusions involve TFE3, the product of which is a transcription factor related to the proto-oncogene product c-myc. Since 2005, various fusions between the androgen-regulated transmembrane protease serine 2 (TMPRSS2), or the solute carrier family 45 member 3 (SLC45A3) genes, on one hand, and E twenty-six (ETS) transcription factors, on the other hand, have been discovered in prostate cancer. The most common fusion, TMPRSS2-ERG, a recurrent and highly prostate cancer-specific event, is indeed present in approximately 50% of prostate-specific antigen (PSA)-screened localized prostate cancers and in 15-35% of population-based cohorts. TMPRSS2-ERG translocation is probably an early event in prostate cancer that is subsequently selected during malignant transformation (Casey et al. 2012).

The observation of gene fusions in common epithelial carcinoma is still scarce. One reason is that previously identified aberrations in hematological malignancies have been identified by karyotyping, and candidate translocations followed up later by further molecular techniques. Karyotyping carcinomas has not been as feasible. The chromosome quality in epithelial neoplasms is particularly poor, often yielding only partial and poor quality karyotypes, leading to inaccurate analysis. Further, clonal heterogeneity due to the presence of cytogenetically unrelated clones, seen in less than 5% of leukemias, lymphomas, and mesenchymal tumors, but in up to 80% of epithelial carcinomas, renders epithelial tumors uniquely problematic in terms of identifying causal aberrations and gene fusions.

In a study involving all of the more than 450 recurrent balanced aberrations documented from more than 45,000 cytogenetically characterized human neoplasms from different tissue types (Mitelman et al. 2004) it was noted that the number of fusion genes as well as the broader subset of rearranged genes in each tumor category were "strictly proportional" to the total number of cases with an abnormal karyotype. In other words, since the incidence of recurrent chromosomal abnormalities, including gene fusions, in different tumor types is "simply a function of the number of cases with an abnormal karyotype", fewer recurrent gene fusions observed in epithelial neoplasms is simply because far fewer accurately determined abnormal karyotypes have been documented from epithelial tumors, and not due to any fundamental tissue-specific differences. This led to the hypothesis that "cytogenetic aberrations resulting in deregulated or rearranged genes may be of greater importance as an initial step in epithelial tumorigenesis than generally believed". Another profound speculation made by the authors is that "the epithelial tumors are characterized by numerous but individually rare, pathogenetically important gene rearrangements that have not yet been identified". Most gene fusions found in solid tumors are listed in Table 1.

Table 1. Gene fusions in solid tumors

Tumor type	Fusion gene
Aggressive midline carcinoma	BRD4-NUT (t(15;19)(q14;p13))
	BRD3-NUT (t(15;9)(q14;q34))
Alveolar soft part sarcoma (soft tissue tumor)	ASPSCR1–TFE3 (t(X;17)(p11;q25))
Rhabdomyosarcoma (soft tissue tumor)	PAX3–FOXO1 (t(2;13)(q35;q14))
	PAX7–FOXO1 (t(1;13)(p36;q14))
	PAX3–NCOA1 (t(2;2)(p23;q36)),
	PAX3–FOXO4 (t(X;2)(q13;q36))
	DUX4-EWSR1 (t(4;22)(q35;q12))

Table 1. (Continued)

Tumor type	Fusion gene
Aneurysmal bone cysts (soft tissue tumor)	THRAP3-USP6 (t(1;17)(p34;p13)) CNBP-USP6 (t(3;17)(q21;p13)) OMD-USP6 (t(9;17)(q22;p13)) CDH11-USP6 (t(16;17)(q21-q22;p13)) COL1A1-USP6 (t(17;17)(p13;q21))
Angiomatoid fibrous histiocytoma (soft tissue tumor)	EWSR1-ATF1 (t(12;22)(q13;q12)) FUS–ATF1 (t(12;16)(q13;p11)) EWSR1–CREB1 (t(2;22)(q33;q12))
Astrocytoma	GOPC-ROS1 (del(6)(q21q21))
Breast carcinoma, secretory	ETV6-NTRK3 (t(12;15)(p13;q25))
Breast cancer (MCF-7 or MDA-MB-175 cell lines)	BCAS4-BCAS3 (t(17;20)(q23;q13)) (MCF-7 cell line) TBL1XR1-RGS17 (t(3;6)(q26;q25)) (MCF-7 cell line) ODZ4-NRG1 (dic(8;11)(p12;q14) and t(8;11)(p12;q14)) (MDA-MB-175 cell line)
Breast cancer	MAGI3-AKT3
Chondroid lipoma of soft tissue (soft tissue tumor)	C11orf95-MKL2 (t(11,16)(q13;p12-13))
Clear cell sarcoma (soft tissue tumor)	EWSR1-ATF1 (t(12;22)(q13;q12)) EWSR1-CREB1 (t(2;22)(q34;q12))
Congenital fibrosarcoma (soft tissue tumor)	ETV6–NTRK3 (t(12;15)(p13;q25))
Dermatofibrosarcoma protuberans (soft tissue tumor):	COL1A1–PDGFB (t(17;22)(q22;q13) and der(22)t(17;22))
Giant cell fibrosarcoma (soft tissue tumor)	COL1A1–PDGFB (t(17;22)(q22;q13))
Desmoplastic small round cell tumor (soft tissue tumor)	EWSR1-WT1 (t(11;22)(p13;q12)) EWSR1-ERG (t(21;22)(q22;q12)) EWSR1-PATZ1 (inv(22)(q12q12))
Endometrial stromal sarcoma (soft tissue tumor)	JAZF1–SUZ12 (t(7;17)(p15;q21)) JAZF1-PHF1 (t(6;7)(p21;p15)) EPC1-PHF1 (t(6;10)(p21;p11))
Ewing sarcoma/PNET (soft tissue tumor)	EWSR1-FLI1 (t(11;22)(q24;q12)) EWSR1-NFATC2 (t(20;22)(q13;q12)) EWSR1-FEV (t(2;22)(q33;q12)) EWSR1-ETV1 (t(7;22)(p22;q12)) EWSR1-E1AF (t(17;22)(q12;q12)) EWSR1-SP3 (t(17;22)(q31;q12)) EWSR1-ERG (t(21;22)(q22;q12)) EWSR1-POU5F1 (t(6;22)(p21;q12)) FUS–ERG (t(16;21)(p11;q22)) EWSR1-PATZ1 (inv(22)(q12q12)) FUS-FEV (t(2;16)(q35;p11)) EWSR1-ETV4 (t(17;22)(q21;q12))
Extraskeletal myxoid chondrosarcoma (soft tissue tumor)	EWSR1-NR4A3 (t(9;22)(q22;q12)) TAF2N–NR4A3 (t(9;17)(q22;q11)) TCF12-NR4A3 (t(9;15)(q22;q21)) TAF15-NR4A3 (t(9;17)(q31;q12)) TFG–NR4A3 (t(3;9)(q12;q22)) EWSR1-CHN1 (t(9;22)(q22–31;q11-12))
Tenosynovial giant cell tumor (soft tissue tumor)	COL6A3-CSF1 (t(1;2)(p13;q37))

Tumor type	Fusion gene
Hibernoma (soft tissue tumor):	C11orf95-MKL2 (t(11,16)(q13;p12-13))
Lipoma (soft tissue tumor)	HMGA2-LPP (t(3;12)(q27-q28;q13-q15))
	HMGA2-LHFP (t(12;13)(q13–15;q12))
Low-grade fibromyxoid sarcoma (soft tissue tumor)	FUS–CREB3L2 (t(7;16)(q33–34;p11))
	FUS–CREB3L1 (t(11;16)(p11;p11))
Kidney carcinoma	MALAT1-TFEB (t(6;11)(p21;q12-q13))
	ASPSCR1-TFE3 (der(X)t(X;17)(p11;q25))
	PRCC-TFE3 (t(X;1)(p11.2;q21))
	CLTC-TFE3 (t(X;17)(p11.2;q23))
	NONO-TFE3 (inv(X)(p11.2;q12))
	SFPQ-TFE3 (t(X;1)(p11;p34))
Inflammatory myofibroblastic tumor (IMT) (soft tissue tumor)	TPM3 – ALK (t(1;2)(q25;q23))
	RANBP2 – ALK (t(2;2)(p23;q13))
	CARS – ALK (t(2;11;2)(p23;p15;q31))
	CLTC – ALK (t(2;17)(q23;q23))
	TPM4 – ALK (t(2;19)(q23;q13))
Pericytoma (soft tissue tumor)	ACTB-GLI1 (t(7;12)(p22;q13))
Lung adenocarcinoma	EML4-ALK (inv(2)(p21p23))
Meningioma	MN1-ETV6 (t(12;22)(p13;q11))
Congenital mesoblastic nephroma (soft tissue tumor)	ETV6-NTRK3 (t(12;15)(p13;q25))
Myoepithelioma	EWSR1-PBX1 (t(1;22)(q23;q12))
Myxoid/round cell liposarcoma (soft tissue tumor)	EWSR1-DDIT3 (t(12;22)(q13;q12))
	FUS–DDIT3 (t(12;16)(q13;p11))
Myxoinflammatory fibroblastic sarcoma (soft tissue tumor)	Ring chromosome amplification of VGLL3
Prostate carcinoma	TMPRSS2-ERG (t(21;21)(q22;q22))
	TMPRSS2-ETV1 (t(7;21)(p21;q22))
	TMPRSS2-ETV4 (t(17;21)(q21;q22.3))
	TMPRSS2-ETV5 (t(3;21)(q27;q22))
	HNRNPA2B1-ETV1 (t(7;7)(p15;p21)
	HERV-K-ETV1 (t(7;22)(p21.2;q11.23))
	C15ORF21-ETV1 (t(7;15)(p21;q21))
	SLC45A3-ETV1 (t(1;7)(q32;p21))
	SLC45A3-ETV5 (t(1;3)(q32;q28))
	SLC45A3-ELK4 (t(1;1)(q32;q32))
	SLC45A3-BRAF (t(1;7)(q32;q34))
	KLK2-ETV4 (t(17;19)(q21;q13))
	CANT1-ETV4 (inv(17;17)(q22;q25))
	ESRP1-RAF (t(3;8)(p25.1;q22.1))
Salivary glands, mucoepidermoid cancer	CRTC1-MAML2 (t(19;11)(p13;q21))
	CRTC3-MAML2 (t(11;15)(q21;q26))
	EWSR1-POU5F1 (t(6;22)(p21;q12))
Salivary glands, pleomorphic adenoma	CTNNB1-PLAG1 (t(3;8)(p21;q12))
	LIFR-PLAG1 (t(5;8)(p13;q12))
	TCEA1-PLAG1 (ins(8)(q12;q11q11))
	FGFR1-PLAG1 (r(8)(p12q12.1))
	CHCHD7-PLAG1 (inv(8)(q12q12))
	HMGA2-FHIT (t(3;12)(q26;p13))
	HMGA2-NFIB (ins(9;12)(p23;q12-15))
	HMGA2-WIF1 (inv(12)(q14q15))

Table 1. (Continued)

Tumor type	Fusion gene
Synovial sarcoma (soft tissue tumor)	SS18–SSX1 (t(X;18)(p11;q11))
	SS18–SSX2 (t(X;18)(p11;q11))
	SS18–SSX4 (t(X;18)(p11;q11))
	SS181–SSX1 (t(X;20)(p11;q13))
Thyroid carcinoma	RET-CCDC6 (inv(10)(q11.2;q21))
	RET-PRKAR1A (t(10;17)(q11.2;q23))
	RET-NCOA4 (inv(10)(q11.2;q11.2))
	RET-GOLGA5 (t(10;14)(q11.2;q32))
	RET-TRIM24 (t(7;10)(q32;q11))
	RET-TRIM33 (t(1;10)(p13;q11))
	RET-KTN1 (t(10;14)(q11.2;q22.1))
	RET-PCM1 (t(8;10)(p21.3;q11.2))
	TFG-NTRK1 (t(1;3)(q21;q11))
	TPM3-NTRK1 (inv(1)(q21q23))
	TPR-NTRK1 (del(1)(q21q23))
	NTRK1-RET (t(1;10)(q21;q11))
	ERC1-RET (t(10;12)(q11;p13))
	HOOK3-RET (t(8;10)(p11.21;q11.2))
	TRIM27-RET (t(6;10)(p21.3;q11.2))
	AKAP9-BRAF (inv(7)(q21-22q34))
	PAX8-PPARG (t(2,3)(q13;p25))
Uterine leiomyoma	HMGA2-CCNB1IP1 (t(12;14)(q14;q11))
	HMGA2-RAD51L1 (t(12;14)(q15;q23-24))

Several gene fusions associated to specific tumor types are currently used for diagnosis, prognosis or therapeutics, based on their accurate detection.

For instance, acute leukemias with the same oncogenetic aberration generally form a clinically and diagnostically homogenous disease entity with comparable prognosis. In consequence, various fusion genes resulting from oncogenetic aberrations in acute leukemias may now be detected by karyotyping, FISH, or RT-PCR analysis.

This is notably the case for BCR-ABL, PML-RARA, TEL-AML1 (the most common fusion event in ALL), E2A-PBX1, MLL-AF4, AML1-ETO and CBFB-MYH11 (Dekking et al. 2010). Translocations EWSR1-FLI1, SS18-SSX1, and PAX3-FOXO1 are used for diagnosis of Ewing family tumors, synovial sarcoma, and alveolar rhabdomyosarcoma, respectively (Gulley and Kaiser-Rogers 2009). The JAZF1-JJAZ1 fusion gene may discriminate between low-grade endometrial stromal sarcomas (ESS), and undifferentiated endometrial sarcomas (UES), the latter representing the most aggressive form. For instance, in an analysis of 20 ESS and 2 UES cases, the JAZF1/JJAZ1 fusion transcript occurred in 80% of analyzed ESS cases and in none of two UES cases (Hrzenjak et al. 2005). Translocation t(11;14)(q13;q32), fusing CCND1 to IGH (the immunoglobulin heavy-chain), resulting in the overexpression of cyclin D1, is the molecular hallmark of mantle cell lymphoma (Vose 2012).

In prostate, TMPRSS2-ERG is now qualified for clinical use.

Table 2. Cancer: common structural chromosomal anomalies involving genes

Deletions		
del(1)(p32p32)	STIL-TAL1	ALL
del(3)(q27q28)	LPP-BCL6	NHL
del(4)(q12q12)	FIP1L1-PDGFRA	CEL
del(6)(q14q22)	SENP6-NKAIN2	T-CLL
del(6)(q21q21)	GOPC-ROS1	Glioblastoma
del(8)(q12q24)	HAS2-PLAG1	Lipoblastoma
del(9)(q34q34)	SET-NUP214	AML, ALL
del(11)(q23q23)	MLL-ARHGEF12	AML
del(11)(q23q23)	MLL-CBL	AML
del(11)(q23q23.3)	MLL-BCL9L	ALL
del(11)(q23q24.2)	MLL-TIRAP	AML
del(11)(q23q24.2)	MLL-DCPS	AML
del(21)(q22q22)	TMPRSS2-ERG	Prostate cancer
Non-reciprocal translocations		
der(5)t(5;9)(q35;q34)	SQSTM1-NUP214	ALL
der(18)t(3;18)(p21;q21)	MALT1-MAP4	NHL
der(X)t(X;17)(p11;q25)	ASPSCR1-TFE3	Alveolar soft part sarcoma
Dicentric aberrations (dic)		
dic(8;11)(p12;q14)	ODZ4-NRG1	Breast cancer
dic(9;12)(p13;p12)	PAX5-SLCO1B3	ALL
dic(9;12)(p13;p13)	PAX5-ETV6	ALL, CML, NHL
dic(9;18)(p13;q11)	PAX5-ZNF521	ALL
dic(9;20)(p11-13;q11)	PAX5-ASXL1	ALL
Insertions		
ins(3;3)(q26;q21q26)	RPN1-EVI1	MDS, AML, CML
ins(4;11)(q21;q23q23)	AFF1-DSCAML1	ALL
ins(5;11)(q31;q13q23)	MLL-AFF4	ALL
ins(8)(q12;q11q11)	TCEA1-PLAG1	Salivary gland, pleomorphic adenoma
ins(8;21)(q22;q22q22)	RUNX1-RUNX1T1	AML
ins(9;4)(q33;q12q25)	CDK5RAP2-PDGFRA	CEL
ins(9;12)(p23;q12q15)	HMGA2-NFIB	Salivary gland, pleomorphic adenoma
ins(10;11)(p12;q23q13)	MLL-MLLT10	AML, AML[t], ALL
ins(10;11)(p12;q23)	MLL-NEBL	AML
ins(11;9)(q23;q34)	MLL-FNBP1	AML
ins(11;17)(q23;q21)	MLL-ACACA	AML
ins(11;19)(q23;p13.2)	MLL-VAV	AML
ins(11;X)(q23;q28q13.1)	MLL-FLNA	AML
ins(12;8)(p11;p11p22)	FGFR1OP2-FGFR1	EMS 8p11
ins(15;17)(q22;q21q21)	PML-RARA	AML
ins(16)(q22p13p13)	CBFB-MYH11	AML, CML, MDS
ins(21;8)(q22;q13q22)	RUNX1-RUNX1T1	AML

Table 2. (Continued)

Insertions		
ins(21;8)(q22;q21q22)	RUNX1-RUNX1T1	AML
ins(21;8)(q22;q22q22)	RUNX1-RUNX1T1	AML
ins(21;22)(q22;q12q12)	EWSR1-ERG	Ewing tumor/PNET
ins(22;9)(q11;q34q34)	BCR-ABL1	CML
ins(X;11)(q24;q23)	MLL-SEPT6	Pediatric AML
Inversions		
inv(1)(q21q23)	TPM3-NTRK1	Papillary thyroid carcinoma
inv(1)(q21q31)	TPM3-TPR	Papillary thyroid carcinoma
inv(1)(q23q31)	TPR-NTRK1	Papillary thyroid carcinoma
inv(2)(p21p23)	EML4-ALK	NSCLC
inv(2)(p23;q11-13)	RANBP2-ALK	IMT
inv(2)(p23q35)	ATIC-ALK	ALCL, IMT
inv(3)(q21q26)	RPN1-EVI1	AML, CML, MDS
inv(6)(p21q21)	HMGA1-LAMA4	Pulmonary chondroid hamartoma
inv(7)(p15q34)	TRB@-HOXA10	T-ALL, NHL
inv(7)(p15q34)	TRB@-HOXA9	T-ALL, NHL
inv(7)(p15q34)	TRB@-HOXA11	T-ALL, NHL
inv(7)(q21-22;q34)	AKAP9-BRAF	Papillary thyroid adenocarcinoma
inv(8)(p11q13)	MYST3-NCOA2	AML
inv(8)(q12q12)	CHCHD7-PLAG1	Salivary gland, pleomorphic adenoma
inv(10)(q11q11)	NCOA4-RET	Germ cell tumor (ovary)
inv(10)(q11.2q21)	CCDC6-RET	Papillary thyroid carcinoma
inv(11)(p15q22)	NUP98-DDX10	MDS[t], AML, AML[t]
inv(11)(p15.3q23)	MLL-NRIP3	AML
inv(11)(q13q23)	MLL-FNBP1	AML
inv(11)(q13.4q23)	MLL-C2CD3	AML
inv(11)(q14q23)	MLL-PICALM	AML
inv(11)(q21q23)	MLL-MAML2	T-ALL, AML[t], MDS
inv(11)(q23q23)	MLL-UBE4A	MDS
inv(12)(q14q15)	HMGA2-WIF1	Salivary gland, pleomorphic adenoma
inv(14)(q11q32)	CEBPE-IGH@	B-ALL
inv(14)(q11q32)	IGH@-TRA@	T-ALL
inv(14)(q11q32)	TRA@/TRD@-TCL1A	T-ALL
inv(14)(q11.2q32.31)	BCL11B-TRD@	T-ALL
inv(16)(p13q22)	CBFB-MYH11	AML, CML, MDS
inv(22)(q12q12)	EWSR1-PATZ1	Desmoplastic small round cell tumor, Ewing tumor/PNET
inv(22)(q21q12)	EWSR1-ZSG	Desmoplastic small round cell tumor, Ewing tumor/PNET
inv(X)(p11.2;q12)	NONO-TFE3	Renal cell carcinoma
Ring chromosome		
r(8)(p12q12)	FGFR1-PLAG1	Salivary gland, pleomorphic adenoma

Balanced translocations		
t(1;1)(p36;q41)	DUSP10-PRDM16	AML
t(1;2)(p13;q37)	COL6A3-CSF1	Diffuse-type giant cell tumor of tendon sheath
t(1;2)(p22;p11)	IGK@-BCL10	NHL
t(1;2)(q25;p23)	TPM3-ALK	IMT, ALCL, renal cell carcinoma
t(1;3)(p32;p21)	TAL1-TCTA	T-ALL
t(1;3)(p36;q21)	RPN1-PRDM16	MDS, AML, AML^t, CML, MPD
t(1;3)(p36;q21)	PSMD2-PRDM16	AML, CML
t(1;3)(q21;q11)	TFG-NTRK1	Papillary thyroid carcinoma
t(1;3)(q25;q27)	GAS5-BCL6	NHL
t(1;3)(q32;q27)	SLC45A3-ETV5	Prostate cancer
t(1;3;5)(p36;p21;q33)	WDR48-PDGFRB	CEL
t(1;5)(q21;q33)	TPM3-PDGFRB	CEL
t(1;5)(q21;q33)	PDE4DIP-PDGFRB	MPD associated with eosinophilia
t(1;5;11)(?;q33;p13)	GPIAP1-PDGFRB	CEL
t(1;7)(p32;q34)	TAL1-TRB@	T-ALL
t(1;7)(p34;q34)	LCK-TRB@	T-ALL
t(1;7)(q32;p21)	SLC45A3-ETV1	Prostate cancer
t(1;9)(p34;q34)	SFPQ-ABL1	B-ALL
t(1;9)(q24;q34)	RCSD1-ABL1	B-ALL
t(1;10)(p13;q11)	TRIM33-RET	Papillary thyroid carcinoma
t(1;10)(q21;q11)	RET-NTRK1	Papillary thyroid carcinoma
t(1;11)(p32;q23)	MLL-EPS15	AML, ALL, bilineage or biphenotypic leukemia
t(1;11)(q21;q23)	MLL-MLLT11	AML, ALL
t(1;11)(q24;p15)	NUP98-PRRX1	AML
t(1;12)(p36;p13)	ETV6-MDS2	CML, RAEB
t(1;12)(q21;p13)	ARNT-ETV6	AML
t(1;12)(q25;p13)	ABL2-ETV6	AML, T-ALL
t(1;13)(p36;q14)	PAX7-FOXO1	Alveolar rhabdomyosarcoma
t(1;14)(p22;q32)	BCL10-IGH@	NHL
t(1;14)(p32;q11)	TAL1-TRD@	T-ALL
t(1;14)(p34;q32)	IGH@-LAPTM5	MM
t(1;14)(q21;q32)	BCL9-IGH@	B-ALL, NHL
t(1;14)(q21;q32)	IGH@-FCRL4	MM
t(1;14)(q21;q32)	FCGR2B-IGH@	NHL
t(1;14)(q21-q22;q32)	MUC1-IGH@	NHL
t(1;14)(q25;q32)	IGH@-LHX4	pre-B-ALL, CML
t(1;17)(p34;p13)	THRAP3-USP6	Aneurysmal bone cyst
t(1;19)(q23;p13)	MEF2D-DAZAP1	ALL
t(1;19)(q23;p13)	TCF3-PBX1	ALL, AML, NHL
t(1;21)(p35;q22)	RUNX1-YTHDF2	AML
t(1;21)(p36;q22)	RUNX1-PRDM16	AML^t, MDS
t(1;21)(q21;q22)	RUNX1-ZNF687	AML
t(1;22)(p13;q13)	RBM15-MKL1	AML
t(1;22)(q21;q11)	BCL9-IGL@	NHL
t(1;22)(q23;q12)	EWSR1-PBX1	Myoepithelioma
t(2;2)(p23;q11-q13)	RANBP2 – ALK	IMT
t(2;2)(p23;q36)	PAX3–NCOA1	Alveolar rhabdomyosarcoma

Table 2. (Continued)

t(2;3)(p11-p12;q27)	IGK@-BCL6	NHL
t(2;3)(p23;q21)	TFG-ALK	NHL, NSCLC
t(2;3)(q13;p25)	PAX8-PPARG	Follicular thyroid carcinoma, follicular adenoma
t(2;4)(p22;q12)	STRN-PDGFRA	MPD with eosinophilia
t(2;4)(p23;q21)	SEC31A-ALK	IMT
t(2;5)(p21;q33)	SPTBN1-PDGFRB	atypical MPD with eosinophilia
t(2;5)(p23;q35)	NPM1-ALK	NHL, IMT
t(2;7)(p11;q21)	CDK6-IGK@	CLL, NHL
t(2;8)(p11;q24)	IGK@-MYC	B-ALL, NHL
t(2;8)(p11;q24)	IGK@-PVT1	NHL
t(2;8)(p23;p11.2)	MYST3-ASXL2	MDS[t]
t(2;11)(p11;q13)	IGK@-CCND1	NHL
t(2;11)(p23;p15)	CARS-ALK	IMT
t(2;11)(q11;q23)	MLL-AFF3	ALL
t(2;11)(q31;p15)	NUP98-HOXD11	AML
t(2;11)(q31;p15)	NUP98-HOXD13	AML, CML
t(2;11)(q37;q23)	MLL-SEPT2	AML, AML[t], MDS[t]
t(2;12)(p11;p13)	IGK@-CCND2	NHL
t(2;12)(q37;q14)	HMGA2-CXCR7	Lipoma
t(2;13)(q35-q36;q14)	PAX3-FOXO1	Alveolar rhabdomyosarcoma
t(2;14)(p13;q32)	BCL11A-IGH@	CLL, ALL, NHL, AML
t(2;16)(q35;p11)	FUS-FEV	Ewing family tumor
t(2;17)(p23;q23)	CLTC-ALK	NHL, IMT
t(2;17)(p23;q25)	RNF213-ALK	NHL
t(2;18)(p11;q21.3)	IGK@-BCL2	CLL/SLL, NHL
t(2;18)(p11;q21)	IGK@-KDSR	NHL
t(2;18)(q11.2;q21.33)	AFF3-BCL2	NHL
t(2;19)(p11-p12;q13)	IGK@-BCL3	CLL, NHL
t(2;19)(p23;p13.1)	TPM4-ALK	NHL, IMT, SCC
t(2;21)(q11;q22)	RUNX1-AFF3	T-ALL
t(2;22)(p23;q11.2)	CLTCL1-ALK	NHL
t(2;22)(p23;q11.2-q12)	MYH9-ALK	NHL
t(2;22)(q31;q12)	EWSR1-SP3	Ewing tumor/PNET, undifferentiated small round cell tumor
t(2;22)(q33-q35;q12)	EWSR1-FEV	Ewing tumor/PNET
t(2;22)(q33;q12)	EWSR1-CREB1	Angiomatoid fibrous histiocytoma, clear cell sarcoma
t(3;3)(q21;q26)	RPN1-EVI1	MDS, AML, CML
t(3;3)(q21;q26)	C3ORF27-EVI1	AML
t(3;3)(q25;q27)	MBNL1-BCL6	NHL
t(3;3)(q27;q27)	BCL6-ST6GAL1	NHL
t(3;3)(q27;q28)	EIF4A2-BCL6	NHL
t(3;3)(q27;q29)	TFRC-BCL6	NHL
t(3;4)(q27;p13)	RHOH-BCL6 (and BCL6-RHOH)	NHL
t(3;5)(p21-25;q31-35)	GOLGA4-PDGFRB	CEL

t(3;5)(p21;q33)	RBM6-CSF1R	AML
t(3;5)(p24;q35)	NSD1-ANKRD28	AML
t(3;5)(q25;q34)	NPM1-MLF1	MDS, AML, CML
t(3;5;11)(p25;q35;p15)	ANKRD28-NUP98	MDS, AML
t(3;6)(q26;q25)	TBL1XR1-RGS17	Breast cancer (MCF7 cell line)
t(3;6)(q27;p12)	HSP90AB1-BCL6	NHL
t(3;6)(q27;p21)	PIM1-BCL6 and BCL6-PIM1	NHL
t(3;6)(q27;p21)	SFRS3-BCL6	NHL
t(3;6)(q27;p22)	BCL6-HIST1H4I	NHL
t(3;6)(q27;q15)	BCL6-SNHG5	NHL
t(3;7)(q27;p12-13)	IKZF1-BCL6	NHL
t(3;7)(q27;q32)	BCL6-FRA7H	NHL
t(3;8)(q27;q24.1)	BCL6-MYC	NHL
t(3;8)(p21;q12)	PLAG1-CTNNB1	Salivary gland, pleomorphic adenoma
t(3;9)(p14;p13)	PAX5-FOXP1	ALL
t(3;9)(q12;q31)	TFG-NR4A3	Extraskeletal myxoid chondrosarcoma
t(3;9)(q27;p11)	BCL6-GRHPR	NHL
t(3;9)(q27;p24)	DMRT1-BCL6	NHL
t(3;11)(p21;q23)	NCKIPSD-MLL	AML[t], ALL
t(3;11)(p21.3;q23)	MLL-DCP1A	ALL
t(3;11)(p24;p15)	NUP98 TOP2B	AML
t(3;11)(q12.2;p15.4)	NUP98-LNP1	T-ALL
t(3;11)(q21;q23)	MLL-EEFSEC	AML
t(3;11)(q25;q23)	MLL-GMPS	AML[t], AML
t(3;11)(q27;q23)	BCL6-POU2AF1	NHL, ALL
t(3;11)(q28;q23)	MLL-LPP	AML[t]
t(3;11)(q29;p15)	NUP98-IQCG	Bi-phenotypic acute T-lymphoid/myeloid leukemia
t(3;12)(p14;q15)	HMGA2-FHIT	Salivary gland, pleomorphic adenoma
t(3;12)(q26;p13)	ETV6-EVI1	MDS, AML, CML
t(3;12)(q27;p13)	GAPDH-BCL6	NHL
t(3;12)(q27;q12)	BCL6-LRMP	NHL
t(3;12)(q27;q15)	HMGA2-LPP	Soft tissue chondroma, parosteal lipoma, pulmonary chondroid hamartoma
t(3;12)(q27;q23)	BCL6-NACA	NHL
t(3;13)(q27;q14)	LCP1-BCL6	NHL
t(3;14)(p14;q32)	IGH@-FOXP1	NHL
t(3;14)(q27;q32)	BCL6-IGH@	NHL
t(3;14)(q27;q32)	HSP90AA1-BCL6	NHL
t(3;16)(q27;p11)	IL21R-BCL6	NHL
t(3;16)(q27;p13)	CIITA-BCL6	NHL
t(3;17)(q21;p13)	CNBP-USP6	Aneurysmal bone cysts
t(3;17)(q26;q22)	EVI1-(unknown)	CML, AML
t(3;19)(q27; q13)	BCL6-NAPA	NHL
t(3;21)(q26;q22)	RUNX1-RPL22P1	CML, AML, MDS
t(3;21)(q26;q22)	RUNX1-MDS1	AML[t], MDS[t]

Table 2. (Continued)

t(3;21)(q26;q22)	RUNX1-EVI1	CML, MDS[t], AML, AML[t]
t(3;21)(q27;q22)	TMPRSS2-ETV5	Prostate adenocarcinoma
t(3;22)(q27;q11)	BCL6-IGL@	NHL
t(4;5)(q21;q33)	PRKG2-PDGFRB	Atypical myeloproliferative disorder, systemic mast cell disease
t(4;6)(p15;q22)	SLC34A2-ROS1	NSCLC
t(4;10)(q12;p11)	KIF5B-PDGFRA	MPS with hypereosinophilia
t(4;11)(p12;q23)	MLL-FRYL	T-ALL, AML[t]
t(4;11)(q21-q23;p15)	NUP98-RAP1GDS1	T-ALL
t(4;11)(q21;q23)	MLL-AFF1	ALL, AML
t(4;11)(q21;q23)	MLL-SEPT11	atypical CML, ALL
t(4;11)(q35;q23)	MLL-SORBS2	AML
t(4;12)(p16;p13)	ETV6-FGFR3	Peripheral T-cell lymphoma
t(4;12)(q11;p13)	CHIC2-ETV6	AML, ALL
t(4;12)(q12;p13)	ETV6-PDGFRA	MPD with eosinophilia
t(4;14)(p14;q32)	IGH@-RHOH	MM
t(4;14)(p16.3;q32.3)	IGH@-FGFR3	MM
t(4;14)(p16;q32)	IGH@-WHSC1	MM, plasma cell leukemia
t(4;16)(q26;p13)	IL2-TNFRSF17	T-cell lymphoma of the small intestine
t(4;17)(q12;q21)	FIP1L1-RARA and RARA-FIP1L1	JMML
t(4;19)(q35;q13)	CIC-DUX4	Ewing-like sarcoma
t(4;21)(q31;q22)	RUNX1-SH3D19	AML
t(4;22)(q12;q11.2)	BCR-PDGFRA	MPD, atypical CML
t(4;22)(q35;q12)	DUX4-EWSR1	Embryonal rhabdomyosarcoma
t(5;6)(q32-q33;q22)	CD74-ROS1	NSCLC
t(5;7)(q31;q34)	FCHSD1-BRAF	Congenital melanocytic nevus
t(5;7)(q33;q11.2)	HIP1-PDGFRB	CMML with eosinophilia
t(5;7)(q35.1;q21)	CDK6-TLX3	ALL
t(5;8)(p13;q12)	LIFR-PLAG1	Salivary gland, pleomorphic adenoma
t(5;9)(q14.1;p24.1)	SSBP2-JAK2	Pre-B-ALL
t(5;9)(q31-q32;p22-p24.3)	KANK1-PDGFRB	Myeloid neoplasm with severe thrombocythemia
t(5;9)(q33;q22)	ITK-SYK	PTCL
t(5;10)(q33;q21)	CCDC6-PDGFRB	Atypical CML, MPD with eosinophilia
t(5;11)(q12;q23)	MLL-CENPK	AML
t(5;11)(q31;q23)	MLL-AFF4	ALL
t(5;11)(q31;q23)	MLL-ARHGAP26	ALL, JMML, AML, AML[t], CML
t(5;11)(q33;p13)	CAPRIN1-PDGFRB	Chronic MPD with eosinophilia
t(5;11)(q35;p15.5)	NUP98-NSD1 and NSD1-NUP98	AML
t(5;12)(q31;p13)	ETV6-ACSL6	AML, MDS, AEL

t(5;12)(q33;p13)	ERC1-PDGFRB	Myeloproliferative/myelodysplastic syndrome (intermediate between CML and CMML) with eosinophilia)
t(5;12)(q33;p13)	ETV6-PDGFRB	CMML
t(5;12)(q33;q14)	HMGA2-EBF1	Lipoma
t(5;12)(q33;q24)	GIT2-PDGFRB	Chronic MPD with eosinophilia
t(5;14)(q31;q32)	IGH@-IL3	ALL
t(5;14)(q33;q22)	NIN-PDGFRB	Chronic MPD with eosinophilia
t(5;14)(q33;q32)	PDGFRB-CCDC88C	Atypical CML
t(5;14)(q33;q32)	TRIP11-PDGFRB	AML
t(5;14)(q35;q11)	RANBP17-TRD@	ALL
t(5;14)(q35;q11)	TRD@-NKX2-5	T-ALL
t(5;14)(q35;q11)	TRD@-TLX3	T-ALL
t(5;14)(q35;q32)	TLX3-BCL11B	T-ALL
t(5;14)(q35.1;q32.2)	BCL11B-NKX2-5	T-ALL
t(5;15)(q33;q15)	TP53BP1-PDGFRB	CEL
t(5;16)(q33;p13)	NDE1-PDGFRB	CML
t(5;17)(q33;p11.2)	SPECC1-PDGFRB	JMML with eosinophilia
t(5;17)(q33;p11.2)	PDGFRB-CYTSB	JMML
t(5;17)(q33;p13)	RABEP1-PDGFRB	CML
t(5;17)(q33-34;q11.2)	MYO18A-PDGFRB	Eosinophilia- associated atypical myeloproliferative neoplasm – Eos-MPN
t(5;17)(q34;q21)	NPM1-RARA	AML
t(5;21)(q13;q22)	RUNX1-(unknown)	AML, MDS
t(6;7)(p21;p15)	JAZF1-PHF1	Endometrial stromal sarcoma
t(6;7)(q23;q34)	TRB@-MYB	T-ALL
t(6;7)(q23;q36)	MYB-MNX1	AML
t(6;8)(q27;p12)	FGFR1OP-FGFR	EMS
t(6;9)(p23;q34)	DEK-NUP214	AML, MDS
t(6;9)(q22–q24;p21–p23)	MYB-NFIB	Breast and salivary glands adenoid cystic carcinoma
t(6;10)(p21;p11)	EPC1-PHF	Endometrial stromal sarcoma
t(6;10)(p21.3;q11.2)	TRIM27-RET	Papillary thyroid carcinoma
t(6;11)(p21;q12-q13)	MALAT1-TFEB	Renal cell carcinoma
t(6;11)(q12;q23)	MLL-SMAP1	AML
t(6;11)(q21;q23)	MLL-FOXO3	AML^t
t(6;11)(q24;p15)	NUP98-CCDC28A	AML
t(6;11)(q27;q23)	MLL-MLLT4	AML, AML^t, ALL
t(6;12)(q23;p13)	ETV6-STL	B-ALL
t(6;14)(p21;q23-24)	HMGA1-RAD51L1	Pulmonary chondroid hamartoma, uterine leiomyoma
t(6;14)(p21;q32)	IGH@-CCND3	MM, NHL
t(6;14)(p22;q32)	IGH@-ID4	BCP-ALL
t(6;14)(p25;q32)	IGH@-IRF4	MM
t(6;22)(p21;q11)	IGL@-CCND3	MM

Table 2. (Continued)

t(6;22)(p21;q12)	EWSR1-POU5F1	Undifferentiated osteosarcoma, mucoepidermoid carcinoma of the salivary glands, hidradenoma
t(7;7)(p15;p21)	HNRPA2B1-ETV1	Prostate cancer
t(7;7)(p15;q34)	TRB@-HOXA10	T-ALL, NHL
t(7;8)(q21;q12)	COL1A2-PLAG1	Lipoblastoma
t(7;8)(q21;q12)	HAS2-PLAG1	Lipoblastoma
t(7;8)(q34;p11)	TRIM24-FGFR1	AML, EMS
t(7;9)(q11;p13)	PAX5-ELN	B-ALL
t(7;9)(q34;q32)	TRB@-TAL2	T-ALL
t(7;9)(q34;q34)	NOTCH1-TRB@	T-ALL
t(7;10)(q34;q11)	TRIM24-RET	Papillary thyroid carcinoma
t(7;10)(q34;q24)	TLX1-TRB@	T-ALL
t(7;11)(p15;p15)	NUP98-HOXA9	AML
t(7;11)(p15;p15)	NUP98-HOXA11	AML, CML, JMML
t(7;11)(p15;p15)	NUP98-HOXA13	AML, MDS
t(7;11)(p22.1;q23)	MLL-TNRC18	ALL
t(7;11)(q21;q23)	CDK6-MLL	ALL
t(7;11)(q34;p13)	TRB@-LMO2	T-ALL
t(7;11)(q34;p15)	TRB@-LMO1	T-ALL
t(7;12)(p22;q13)	ACTB-GLI1	Pericytoma
t(7;12)(q34;p13)	TRB@-CCND2	T-ALL
t(7;12)(q36;p13)	MNX1-ETV6	AML, RAEB^t, ALL
t(7;14)(p14;q32)	TRG@-IGH@	NHL
t(7;14)(q21;q32)	CDK6-IGH@	CLL
t(7;14)(q21;q32)	IGH@-ERVWE1	CLL
t(7;14)(q34;q11)	TRA@-TRB@	ALL
t(7;14)(q35;q32.1)	TRB@-TCL1A	T-ALL
t(7;15)(p21;q21)	C15ORF21-ETV1	Prostate cancer
t(7;16)(q33;p11)	FUS-CREB3L2	Low grade fibromyxoid sarcoma
t(7;17)(p15;q11-q21)	JAZF1-SUZ12	Endometrial stromal cell sarcoma
t(7;17)(p15;q23)	MSI2-HOXA9	CML
t(7;19)(q34;p13)	LYL1-TRB@	T-ALL
t(7;21)(p21;q22)	TMPRSS2-ETV1	Prostate cancer
t(7;21)(p22;q22)	RUNX1-USP42	AML
t(7;22)(p21;q12)	ETV1-EWSR1	Ewing's tumors/PNET
t(7;22)(q21;q11)	IGL@-CDK6	CLL
t(8;9)(p12;q23)	CEP110-FGFR1 and FGFR1-CEP110	EMS, NHL
t(8;9)(p22;p24)	PCM1-JAK2	atypical CML, CEL, ALL, NHL
t(8;9)(q24;p13)	MYC-ZBTB5	NHL
t(8;9)(q24;p13)	MYC-ZCCHC7	NHL
t(8;10)(p22;q11)	PCM1-RET	Papillary thyroid carcinoma
t(8;11)(p11;p15)	NUP98-WHSC1L1	AML
t(8;11)(p12;q14)	ODZ4-NRG1	Breast cancer
t(8;12)(p11-p12;q15)	CPSF6-FGFR1	EMS
t(8;12)(q13;p13)	ETV6-NCOA2	ALL, AML
t(8;12)(q21;q22)	BTG1-MYC	CLL

t(8;12)(q22;q15)	COX6C-HMGA2	Uterine leiomyoma
t(8;13)(p12;q12)	ZMYM2-FGFR1	AML, NHL
t(8;14)(q11;q32)	IGH@-CEBPD	ALL, rarely CML
t(8;14)(q24;q11)	TRA@-MYC	ALL
t(8;14)(q24;q11)	TRD@-PVT1	ALL
t(8;14)(q24;q32)	MYC-IgH@	B-ALL, NHL
t(8;16)(p11;p13)	MYST3-CREBBP	AML
t(8;17)(p12;q11)	MYO18A-FGFR1	EMS
t(8;19)(p11;p13)	MYST3-(unknown)	AML
t(8;19)(q24;q13.1)	MYC-BCL3	AML
t(8;20)(p11;q13)	MYST3-NCOA3	AML
t(8;21)(q21-q22;q22)	RUNX1-RUNX1T1	AML, CML
t(8;21)(q23;q22)	ZFPM2-RUNX1	RAEB
t(8;21)(q24;q22)	RUNX1-TRPS1	T-ALL, AML
t(8;22)(p11;q13)	MYST3-EP300	AML
t(8;22)(p12;q11)	BCR-FGFR1	CML, EMS
t(8;22)(p21;q12)	PPP2R2A-CHEK2	Childhood teratoma
t(8;22)(q24;q11)	IGL@-MYC	B-ALL, NHL, MM
t(8;22)(q24;q11)	IGL@-PVT1	ALL, MM
t(9;9)(p21;p21)	MTS2-MTS1	pediatric ALL
t(9;9)(q34;q34)	NUP214-ABL1	T-ALL
t(9;9)(q34;q34)	SET-NUP214	Acute undifferentiated leukemia
t(9;10)(q34;q22.3)	ZMIZ1-ABL1	B-ALL
t(9;11)(p22;p15)	NUP98-PSIP1	AML, CML-BC
t(9;11)(p22;q23)	MLL-MLLT3	AML, AML^t, ALL
t(9;11)(q34;p15)	NUP98-PRRX2	AML^t
t(9;11)(q34;q23)	MLL-DAB2IP	AML
t(9;11)(q34;q23)	MLL-FNBP1	AML
t(9;12)(p13;p13)	PAX5-ETV6	ALL, CML, NHL
t(9;12)(p22-p23;q14)	HMGA2-NFIB	Lipoma, mixed salivary gland adenoma
t(9;12)(p24;p13)	JAK2-ETV6	T-ALL, B-ALL, CML
t(9;12)(q22;p12)	ETV6-SYK	MDS
t(9;12)(q34;p13)	ETV6-ABL1	ALL, AML, CML
t(9;14)(p13;q32)	IGH@-PAX5	B-cell lymphoproliferative disorders
t(9;14)(p21;q11)	TRA@-CDKN2A	ALL
t(9;14)(q34;q32)	EML1-ABL1	T-ALL
t(9;15)(p13;q24)	PAX5-PML	ALL
t(9;15)(q22;q21)	TCF12-NR4A3	Extraskeletal myxoid chondrosarcoma
t(9;17)(q22;p13)	OMD-USP6	Aneurysmal bone cyst
t(9;17)(q31;q12)	TAF15-NR4A3	Extraskeletal myxoid chondrosarcoma
t(9;18)(p13;q11.2)	PAX5-ZNF521	ALL
t(9;22)(p24;q11.2)	BCR-JAK2	CML
t(9;22)(q22;q12)	EWSR1-NR4A3	Extraskeletal myxoid chondrosarcoma

Table 2. (Continued)

t(9;22)(q34;q11)	BCR-ABL1	CML, ALL, AML, Burkitt lymphoma/leukemia, DLBCL, MM, MDS
t(10;11)(p11.2;q23)	MLL-ABI1	AML
t(10;11)(p13;q21)	PICALM-MLLT10 and MLLT10-PICALM	T-ALL, AML
t(10;11)(p12;q23)	MLL-MLLT10	AML, AML^t, ALL
t(10;11)(q21;q23)	MLL-TET1	AML
t(10;11)(q23;p15)	NUP98-HHEX	AML^t
t(10;11)(q25;p15)	NUP98–ADD3	T-ALL with biphenotypic characteristics
t(10;12)(q11;p13)	ERC1-RET	Papillary thyroid carcinoma
t(10;12)(q24;p13)	ETV6-GOT1	CMML, MDS
t(10;14)(q11.2;q22.1)	KTN1-RET	Papillary thyroid carcinoma
t(10;14)(q11;q32)	RET-GOLGA5	Papillary thyroid carcinoma
t(10;14)(q24;q11)	TLX1-TRA@/TRD@	T-ALL
t(10;14)(q24;q32)	IGH@-NFKB2	B-NHL
t(10;16)(q22;p13)	MYST4-CREBBP	AML, MDS*
t(10;17)(q11;q24)	PRKAR1A-RET	Papillary thyroid carcinoma
t(11;11)(p15;q22)	NUP98-DDX10	MDS, MDS^t, AML, AML^t, CML
t(11;11)(q13;q23)	MLL-ARHGEF17	AML
t(11;11)(q14;q23)	PICALM-MLL	AML
t(11;11)(q23;q23)	CBL-MLL	AML
t(11;11)(q23;q23)	MLL-ARHGEF12	AML
t(11;11)(q23;q23)	MLL-MLL	AML, ALL
t(11;12)(p15;p13)	NUP98-KDM5A	AML
t(11;12)(p15;q13)	NUP98-HOXC11	AML
t(11;12)(p15;q13)	NUP98-HOXC13	AML
t(11;12)(q23;q13)	MLL-SARNP	AML
t(11;14)(p13;q11)	TRA@/TRD@-LMO2	T-ALL
t(11;14)(p15;q11)	TRA@/TRD@-LMO1	T-ALL
t(11;14)(q13;q32)	CCND1-IGH@	NHL
t(11;14)(q23;q23)	MLL-GPHN	AML, AML^t
t(11;14)(q23;q32)	IGH@ DDX6	ALL, B-NHL
t(11;14)(q23;q32)	IGH@-PAFAH1B2	NHL
t(11;14)(q23;q32)	IGH@-PCSK7	Mature B-cell neoplasm
t(11;15)(q21;q26)	CRTC3–MAML2	Salivary gland, mucoepidermoid carcinoma
t(11;15)(q23q;q21)	MLL-UBE4A	MDS
t(11;15)(q23;q14)	MLL-CASC5	AML, AML^t
t(11;15)(q23;q15)	MLL-ZFYVE19	AML
t(11;16)(p11;p11)	FUS-CREB3L1	Low-grade fibromyxoid tumor
t(11;16)(q13;p13)	C11orf95-MKL2	Chondroid lipoma of soft tissue, hibernoma
t(11;16)(q23;p13)	MLL-CREBBP	MDS^t, AML^t, T-ALL, CML

t(11;17)(p15;p13)	NUP98-PHF23	AML
t(11;17)(q13;q21)	NUMA1-RARA	AML
t(11;17)(q23;p13)	MLL-GAS7	ALL, AML, AML^t
t(11;17)(q23;q12)	MLL-ACACA	AML
t(11;17)(q23;q12)	MLL-LASP1	AML
t(11;17)(q23;q12)	MLL-RARA	AML
t(11;17)(q23;q12)	MLL-MLLT6	AML
t(11;17)(q23;q21)	ZBTB16-RARA and RARA-ZBTB16	AML, APL
t(11;17)(q23;q25)	MLL-SEPT9	AML, AML^t, ALL
t(11;18)(p15;q12)	NUP98-SETBP1	T-ALL
t(11;18)(q22;q21)	BIRC3-MALT1	NHL
t(11;19)(q13;p13)	CCND1-FSTL3	B-CLL
t(11;19)(q21;p13)	MAML2-CRTC1	Clear cell hidradenoma of the skin, Warthin's Tumors
t(11;19)(q23;p13)	MLL-SH3GL1	AML
t(11;19)(q23;p13)	MLL-MYO1F	AML
t(11;19)(q23;p13.1)	MLL-ELL	AML, AML^t, MDS
t(11;19)(q23;p13.3)	MLL-MLLT1	AML, ALL
t(11;19)(q23;p13.3)	MLL-ACER1	ALL
t(11;19)(q23;q13)	MLL-ACTN4	ALL
t(11;20)(p15;q11-q12)	NUP98-TOP1	AML, MDS^t
t(11;20)(q23;q11)	MLL-MAPRE1	ALL
t(11;21)(q13;q22)	RUNX1-MACROD1 and MACROD1-RUNX	AML, CML, MDS
t(11;22)(p13;q12)	EWSR1-WT1	Desmoplastic small round cell tumor
t(11;22)(q13;q11)	IGL@-CCND1	Mature B-cell neoplasm, mantle cell lymphoma
t(11;22)(q23;q11.2)	MLL-SEPT5	AML, T-ALL
t(11;22)(q23;q13)	MLL-EP300	AML^t
t(11;22)(q24;q12)	EWSR1-FLI1	Ewing's tumors/ PNET, giant cell tumor of bone, solid pseudopapillary tumor of the pancreas, rhabdomyosarcoma, desmoplastic small round cell tumor
t(12;12)(p13;q13)	ETV6-BAZ2A	ALL
t(12;13)(p12;q12-14)	ETV6-CDX2	CML, MDS, AML, ALL
t(12;13)(p13;q12)	ETV6-FLT3	ALL, MPD with eosinophilia
t(12;13)(p13;q14)	TTL-ETV6	ALL
t(12;13)(q14;q13)	HMGA2-LHFP	lipoma
t(12;14)(p13;q11)	TRA@-CCND2	T-ALL
t(12;14)(p13;q32)	IGH@-CCND2	NHL variant mantle cell lymphoma
t(12;14)(p13;q32)	IGH@-ETV6	ALL
t(12;14)(q14;q11)	HMGA2-CCNB1IP1	Uterine leiomyoma
t(12;14)(q14;q24)	HMGA2-RAD51L1	Uterine leiomyoma

Table 2. (Continued)

t(12;14)(q23;q32)	IGH@-CHST11	B-CLL
t(12;15)(p13;q25)	ETV6-NTRK3	Congenital fibrosarcoma, congenital mesoblastic nephroma, secretory breast carcinoma, AML
t(12;16)(p13;p13)	LAG3-MYH11	AML
t(12;16)(q13;p11)	FUS-DDIT3	myxoid liposarcoma
t(12;16)(q13;p11.2)	FUS-ATF1	Angiomatoid fibrous histiocytoma, myxoid liposarcoma
t(12;17)(p13;p13)	ETV6-PER1	CMML
t(12;17)(p13;q12)	TAF15-ZNF384	AML, ALL
t(12;19)(p13.3; p13.3)	NOP2-TCF3	ALL
t(12;19)(p13;p13)	TCF3-ZNF384	pro-B-ALL
t(12;21)(p13;q22)	ETV6-RUNX1	B-ALL
t(12;21)(q12;q22)	RUNX1-CPNE8	AML
t(12;22)(p13;q11)	IGL@-CCND2	NHL
t(12;22)(p13;q12)	MN1-ETV6	AML, MDS, meningioma
t(12;22)(p13;q12)	EWSR1-ZNF384	pro-B-ALL, biphenotypic leukemia
t(12;22)(q13;q12)	EWSR1-ATF1	Angiomatoid fibrous histiocytoma, malignant melanoma of soft parts, clear cell sarcoma, malignant lipomatous tumors
t(12;22)(ql3;ql2)	EWSR1-DDIT3	Myxoid liposarcoma
t(14;14)(q11;q32)	IGH@-CEBPE	B-ALL
t(14;14)(q11;q32)	TRA@-CEBPE	ALL
t(14;14)(q11;q32)	IGH@-TRA@	T-cell lymphoma
t(14;14)(q11;q32)	TRA@/TRD@-TCL1A	T-PLL, ALL, AML
t(14;15)(q32;q11-13)	IGH@-BCL8	NHL variant DLBCL
t(14;16)(q32;q23)	IGH@-WWOX	MM
t(14;16)(q32;q23)	IGH@-MAF	MM
t(14;18)(q32;q21)	IGH@-MALT1	NHL variant MALT lymphoma, DLBCL, extranodal marginal zone B-cell lymphoma
t(14;18)(q32;q21)	IGH@-BCL2	NHL variants follicular lymphoma, and DLBCL, CLL, ALL
t(14;19)(q11;q13)	PVRL2-TRA@	Peripheral T-cell lymphoma, angioimmunoblastic T-cell lymphoma
t(14;19)(q32;q13)	IGH@-BCL3	CLL, NHL variant follicular lymphoma
t(14;19)(q32;q13)	IGH@-CEBPA	ALL
t(14;19)(q32;q13)	IGH@-CEBPG	ALL
t(14;19)(q32;q13)	IGH@-EPOR	ALL
t(14;19)(q32;q13)	IGH@-SPIB	NHL variant DLBCL
t(14;20)(q32;q12)	IGH@-MAFB	MM
t(14;20)(q32;q13)	IGH@-CEBPB	ALL
t(14;21)(q11;q22)	TRA@-OLIG2	T-ALL

t(14;22)(q32;q11)	IGH@-IGL@	CLL/SLL, NHL variant DLBCL
t(15;9)(q14;q34)	BRD3-NUT	Lethal carcinoma arising in midline organs of young people
t(15;17)(q24;q21)	PML-RARA and RARA-PML	AML, APL, AML^t, CML
t(15;19)(q14;p13)	BRD4-NUT	Lethal carcinoma arising in midline organs of young people, squamous cell carcinoma
t(16;16)(p13;q22)	CBFB-MYH11	AML, MDS
t(16;17)(q21-q22;p13)	CDH11-USP6	Aneurysmal bone cysts
t(16;21)(p11;q22)	FUS-ERG	AML, CML, Ewing family tumor
t(16;21)(q13;q22)	HERPUD1-ERG	Breast adenocarcinoma, prostate cancer
t(16;21)(q24;q22)	RUNX1-CBFA2T3	MDS, AML AML^t
t(16;22)(q23;q11)	IGL@-WWOX	MM
t(16;22)(q23;q11)	IGL@-MAF	MM
t(17;17)(p13;q21)	COL1A1-USP6	Aneurysmal bone cysts
t(17;17)(q21;q21)	STAT5B-RARA	AML
t(17;17)(q21;q24)	PRKAR1A-RARA	AML
t(17;19)(q21;q13)	KLK2-ETV4	Prostate cancer
t(17;19)(q22;p13)	TCF3-HLF	ALL
t(17;20)(q23;q13)	BCAS3-BCAS4	Breast cancer
t(17;21)(q21;q22)	TMPRSS2-ETV4	Prostate cancer
t(17;22)(q12;q12)	EWSR1-E1AF	Ewing's tumors/PNET
t(17;22)(q21;q12)	EWSR1-ETV4	Ewing's tumors/PNET
t(17;22)(q21-q22;q13)	COL1A1-PDGFB	Dermatofibrosarcoma protuberans, pigmented dermatofibrosarcoma protuberans (Bednar tumor), giant cell fibroblastoma
t(18;22)(q21;q11)	IGL@-BCL2	NHL variants follicular and DLBCL
t(19;19)(p13;q13)	TCF3-TFPT	ALL
t(19;22)(q13;q11)	BCL3-IGL@	CLL, NHL variant follicular lymphoma
t(19;22)(q13;q12)	EWSR1-ZNF444	Myoepithelial carcinoma
t(20;22)(q13;q12)	EWSR1-NFATC2	Clear cell sarcoma
t(21;21)(q22;q22)	TMPRSS2-ERG	Prostate cancer
t(21;22)(q22;q12)	EWSR1-ERG	Ewing's tumors/PNET, desmoplastic small-cell round-cell tumor
t(X;1)(p11;p34)	SFPQ-TFE3	Papillary renal cell carcinoma
t(X;1)(p11.2;q21-q23)	PRCC-TFE3	Papillary renal cell carcinoma
t(X;2)(q11;p23)	MSN-ALK	NHL variant ALCL
t(X;2)(q13;q36)	PAX3–FOXO4	Alveolar rhabdomyosarcoma
t(X;2)(q13;q36)	PAX3-MLLT7	Alveolar rhabdomyosarcoma
t(X;6)(q22;q13-14)	COL4A5-COL12A1	Bone subungual exostosis
t(X;7)(q28;q34)	TRB@-MTCP1	T-ALL
t(X;11)(q13;q23)	MLL-FOXO4 and FOXO4-MLL	AML, T-ALL
t(X;11)(q21;q23)	ARHGAP20-BRWD3	B-CLL

Table 2. (Continued)

t(X;11)(q24;q23)	MLL-SEPT6	AML
t(X;14)(p22;q32)/t(Y;14)(p11;q32)	CRLF2-IGH@	B-ALL
t(X;14)(q28;q11)	TRA@-MTCP1	T-PLL
t(X;17). (p11.2;q23)	CLTC-TFE3	Renal cell carcinoma
t(X;17)(p11.2;q25)	ASPSCR1-TFE3	Renal adenocarcinoma, alveolar soft part sarcoma
t(X;18)(p11;q11)	SS18-SSX1	Synovial sarcoma
t(X;18)(p11;q11)	SS18-SSX2	Synovial sarcoma
t(X;18)(p11;q11)	SS18-SSX4	Synovial sarcoma
t(X;18)(p11;q11)	SYT-SSX2	Synovial sarcoma
t(X;20)(p11;q13)	SS18L1-SSX1	Synovial sarcoma
t(X;21)(p22;q22)	RUNX1-PRDX4	AML
t(X;21)(q25-26; q22)	ELF4-ERG	AML

Table 3. Abbreviations

Abbreviation	Term
AEL	Acute eosinophilic leukemia
AL	Acute leukemia
ALCL	Anaplastic large-cell lymphoma
ALL	Acute lymphocytic leukemia
AML	Acute myelogenous leukemia
AML[t]	Acute myelogenous leukemia (primarily treatment associated)
APL	Acute promyelocytic leukemia
B-ALL	B-cell acute lymphocytic leukaemia
B-CLL	B-cell Lymphocytic leukemia
B-NHL	B-cell Non-Hodgkin Lymphoma
BCC	Basal cell carcinoma
BCP-ALL	B-cell precursor acute lymphoblastic leukemia
CEL	Chronic eosinophilic leukemia
CLL	Chronic lymphatic leukemia
CML	Chronic myeloid leukemia
CMML	Chronic myelomonocytic leukemia
CNS	Central nervous system
DFSP	Dermatofibrosarcoma protuberans
DLBCL	Diffuse large B-cell lymphoma
DLCL	Diffuse large-cell lymphoma
EMS	8p11 myeloproliferative syndrome
FL	Follicular lymphoma
GIST	Gastrointestinal stromal tumour
HL	Hodgkin lymphoma
HNPCC	Hereditary non-polyposis colorectal cancer
IMT	Inflammatory myofibroblastic tumor
JMML	Juvenile myelomonocytic leukemia
MALT	Mucosa-associated lymphoid tissue lymphoma

Abbreviation	Term
MDS	Myelodysplastic syndrome
MDS^t	Myelodysplastic syndrome (primarily treatment associated)
MLCLS	Mediastinal large cell lymphoma with sclerosis
MM	Multiple myeloma
MPD	Myeloproliferative disorder
MPS	Myeloproliferative syndrome
NHL	Non-Hodgkin lymphoma
NK/T	Natural killer T cell
NSCLC	Non small cell lung cancer
PMBL	Primary mediastinal B-cell lymphoma
PNET	Primitive neurectodermal tumors
pre-B All	Pre-B-cell acute lymphoblastic leukaemia
PTCL	Peripheral T-cell lymphoma
RAEB	Refractory anemia with excess blasts
RAEB^t	Refractory anemia with excess blasts (primarily treatment associated)
RCC	Renal cell carcinoma
SCC	Squamous cell carcinoma
SLL	Small lymphocytic lymphoma
T-ALL	T-cell acute lymphoblastic leukemia
T-CLL	T-cell chronic lymphocytic leukaemia
TGCT	Testicular germ cell tumour
T-PLL	T cell prolymphocytic leukaemia

References

Aifantis I, Raetz E, Buonamici S. Molecular pathogenesis of T-cell leukaemia and lymphoma. *Nat Rev Immunol.* 2008 May;8(5):380-90.

Bernt KM, Armstrong SA. Targeting epigenetic programs in MLL-rearranged leukemias. *Hematology Am Soc Hematol Educ Program.* 2011;2011:354-60.

Casey OM, Fang L, Hynes PG, Abou-Kheir WG, Martin PL, Tillman HS, Petrovics G, Awwad HO, Ward Y, Lake R, et al. TMPRSS2- Driven ERG Expression In Vivo Increases Self-Renewal and Maintains Expression in a Castration Resistant Subpopulation. *PLoS One.* 2012;7(7):e41668.

De Braekeleer E, Douet-Guilbert N, Rowe D, Bown N, Morel F, Berthou C, Férec C, De Braekeleer M. ABL1 fusion genes in hematological malignancies: a review. *Eur J Haematol.* 2011 May;86(5):361-71.

Dekking E, van der Velden VH, Böttcher S, Brüggemann M, Sonneveld E, Koning-Goedheer A, Boeckx N, Lucio P, Sedek L, Szczepański T, et al. Detection of fusion genes at the protein level in leukemia patients via the flow cytometric immunobead assay. *Best Pract Res Clin Haematol.* 2010 Sep;23(3):333-45.

Gulley ML, Kaiser-Rogers KA. A rational approach to genetic testing for sarcoma. *Diagn Mol Pathol.* 2009 Mar;18(1):1-10.

Hrzenjak A, Moinfar F, Tavassoli FA, Strohmeier B, Kremser ML, Zatloukal K, Denk H. JAZF1/JJAZ1 gene fusion in endometrial stromal sarcomas: molecular analysis by reverse transcriptase-polymerase chain reaction optimized for paraffin-embedded tissue. *J Mol Diagn.* 2005 Aug;7(3):388-95.

Kantarjian HM, Baccarani M, Jabbour E, Saglio G, Cortes JE. Second-generation tyrosine kinase inhibitors: the future of frontline CML therapy. *Clin Cancer Res.* 2011 Apr 1;17(7):1674-83.

Kumar-Sinha C, Tomlins SA, Chinnaiyan AM. Evidence of recurrent gene fusions in common epithelial tumors. *Trends Mol Med.* 2006 Nov;12(11):529-36.

Lannon CL, Sorensen PH. ETV6-NTRK3: a chimeric protein tyrosine kinase with transformation activity in multiple cell lineages. *Semin Cancer Biol.* 2005 Jun;15(3):215-23.

Mitelman F, Johansson B, Mertens F. Fusion genes and rearranged genes as a linear function of chromosome aberrations in cancer. *Nat Genet.* 2004 Apr;36(4):331-4.

Mitelman F, Johansson B, Mertens F. The impact of translocations and gene fusions on cancer causation. *Nat Rev Cancer.* 2007 Apr;7(4):233-45.

Mrózek K, Bloomfield CD. Clinical significance of the most common chromosome translocations in adult acute myeloid leukemia. *J Natl Cancer Inst Monogr.* 2008;(39):52-7.

Nowell PC, Hungerford DA. Chromosome studies on normal and leukemic human leukocytes. *J Natl Cancer Inst.* 1960 Jul;25:85-109.

Pierotti MA, Santoro M, Jenkins RB, Sozzi G, Bongarzone I, Grieco M, Monzini N, Miozzo M, Herrmann MA, Fusco A, et al.

Rabbitts TH. Chromosomal translocations in human cancer. Nature. 1994 Nov 10;372(6502):143-9. Characterization of an inversion on the long arm of chromosome 10 juxtaposing D10S170 and RET and creating the oncogenic sequence RET/PTC. *Proc Natl Acad Sci U S A.* 1992 Mar 1;89(5):1616-20.

Sugawara E, Togashi Y, Kuroda N, Sakata S, Hatano S, Asaka R, Yuasa T, Yonese J, Kitagawa M, Mano H, et al. Identification of anaplastic lymphoma kinase fusions in renal cancer: Large-scale immunohistochemical screening by the intercalated antibody-enhanced polymer method. *Cancer.* 2012 Sep 15;118(18):4427-36.

Vose JM. Mantle cell lymphoma: 2012 update on diagnosis, risk-stratification, and clinical management. *Am J Hematol.* 2012 Jun;87(6):604-9.

Chapter 3

Gene Amplification in Cancer

Abstract

Amplification - somatically acquired increase in copy number of a restricted region of the genome is a frequent event in most cancers. Integrated genome-wide screens of DNA copy number and gene expression in human cancers have accelerated the rate of discovery of amplified and overexpressed genes. Well-known examples of amplified genes include MYCN in neuroblastoma and ERBB2 in breast cancer. For most of the genes identified as yet, there is increasing evidence of involvement in the development of human cancer.

Introduction

Gene amplification refers to the somatically acquired increase in copy number of a restricted region of the genome that is the underlying genomic mechanism that results in overexpression of a dominantly acting cancer gene. Amplification is a common event in cancer. It may involve a single gene encompassing only a few kilobases or may cover several megabases of DNA and multiple genes. In that latter case, consideration of the pattern of genetic alteration alone is usually insufficient to identify the cancer gene that is being selected for in the amplicon and is contributing to oncogenesis. More information is usually required, including physical mapping of the amplicon in multiple cancers, evidence that amplified genes are accompanied by overexpression in tumors that have the amplicon, correlation of amplification and/or overexpression with clinical outcome data, biological investigations of function and in some cases the efficacy of drugs targeted against the overexpressed proteins.

Gene amplification in human cancer cells generates two cytogenetically identifiable structures: extrachromosomal double minutes (autonomously replicating small circular DNA of genomic origin) and the chromosomal homogeneously staining region (Shimizu et al. 2009).

Although multiple copies of complete chromosomes (aneuploidy) and entire genomes (ploidy) are frequent in malignancies, and clearly increase the copy of genes, these are not generally considered as amplification events and are not included in this chapter. The number of copies of a DNA sequence that constitutes genomic amplification is variously described but generally considered greater than 4 or 5 fold relative to an adjacent non-amplified marker on the same chromosome. In a diploid genome this would be equivalent to more than 8 copies. In some cases, the number of copies may be very high. In some neuroblastoma, hundreds of MYC copies have been detected, while some breast tumors may harbor dozens of ERBB2 copies.

Amplified Genes

Table 1. Genes frequently amplified in cancer

Gene symbol	Gene name	Gene locus	Cancer type
AKT2	V-akt murine thymoma viral oncogene homolog 2	19q13.1-q13.2	ovarian cancer
AR	Androgen receptor	Xq11.2-q12	prostate
ARPC1A	Actin related protein 2/3 complex, subunit 1A, 41kDa	7q22.1	pancreas
AURKA	Aurora kinase A	20q13.2-q13.3	breast esophageal bladder
BCL2L2	BCL2-like 2	14q11.2-q12	lung
CACNA1E	Calcium channel, voltage-dependent, R type, alpha 1E subunit	1q25-q31	Wilms tumor
CCND1	Cyclin D1	11q13	lung, breast, oral, melanoma
CCNE1	Cyclin E1	19q12	esophageal, breast
CDK4	Cyclin-dependent kinase 4	12q14	glioma, sarcoma, breast, melanoma
CDK6	Cyclin-dependent kinase 6	7q21-q22	glioma, myxofibrosarcoma
CHD1L	Chromodomain helicase DNA binding protein 1-like	1q12	liver
CKS1B	CDC28 protein kinase regulatory subunit 1B	1q21.2	breast, multiple myeloma, squamous cell carcinoma, lung cancer
DCUN1D1	DCN1, defective in cullin neddylation 1, domain containing 1	3q26.3	squamous cell carcinoma
DYRK2	Dual-specificity tyrosine-(Y)-phosphorylation regulated kinase 2	12q15	lung, esophageal cancer
E2F3	E2F transcription factor 3	6p22	bladder
EGFR	Epidermal growth factor receptor	7p12	glioma, lung, esophageal, colorectal, breast
EIF5A2	Eukaryotic translation initiation factor 5A2	3q26.2	ovarian, lung
ERBB2	V-erb-b2 erythroblastic leukemia viral oncogene homolog 2, neuro/glioblastoma derived oncogene homolog	17q11.2-q12	gastric, esophageal cancer, breast, ovarian, endometrial, bladder

Gene symbol	Gene name	Gene locus	Cancer type
FADD	Fas (TNFRSF6)-associated via death domain	11q13.3	laryngeal squamous cell carcinoma
FGFR1	Fibroblast growth factor receptor 1	8p11.2-p11.1	rhabdomyosarcoma, breast carcinoma (lobular type)
GATA6	GATA binding protein 6	18q11.1-q11.2	pancreatobiliary
GPC5	Glypican 5	13q32	rhabdomyosarcoma
GRB7	Growth factor receptor-bound protein 7	17q12	breast
JUN	Jun proto-oncogene	1p32-p31	sarcoma
KIT	V-kit Hardy-Zuckerman 4 feline sarcoma viral oncogene homolog	4q11-q12	testicular germ cell cancer, glioblastoma, pediatric osteosarcoma
MAP3K5	Mitogen-activated protein kinase kinase kinase 5	6q22.33	histiocytoma
MDM2	Mdm2, p53 E3 ubiquitin protein ligase homolog	12q14.3-q15	sarcoma, breast cancer, neuroblastoma, lung, glioma
MDM4	Mdm4 p53 binding protein homolog	1q32	retinoblastoma, glioma, osteosarcoma
MED29	Mediator complex subunit 29	19q13.2	pancreatic
MET	Met proto-oncogene (hepatocyte growth factor receptor)	7q31	gastric, lung, glioma
MITF	Microphthalmia-associated transcription factor	3p14.2-p14.1	melanoma
MTDH	Metadherin	8q22.1	breast
MYC	V-myc myelocytomatosis viral oncogene homolog	8q24.21	gastric, prostate cancer, medulloblastoma, breast, colon, lung
MYCL1	V-myc myelocytomatosis viral oncogene homolog 1, lung carcinoma derived	1p34.2	lung
MYCN	V-myc myelocytomatosis viral related oncogene, neuroblastoma derived	2p24.1	neuroblastoma, rhabdomyosarcoma, lung, retinoblastoma, medulloblastoma, Wilms tumor
NCOA3	Nuclear receptor coactivator 3	20q12	breast
NKX2-1	NK2 homeobox 1	14q13	lung
NKX2-8	NK2 homeobox 8	14q13.3	lung
PAK1	P21 protein (Cdc42/Rac)-activated kinase 1	11q13-q14	breast
PAX9	Paired box 9	14q12-q13	lung
PIK3CA	Phosphoinositide-3-kinase alpha polypeptide	3q26.3	ovarian
PPM1D	Protein phosphatase, Mg2+/Mn2+ dependent, 1D	17q23.2	breast
PRKCI	Protein kinase C, iota	3q26.3	squamous cell carcinoma
RAB25	RAB25, member RAS oncogene family	1q22	breast, ovarian

Table 1. (Continued)

Gene symbol	Gene name	Gene locus	Cancer type
REL	V-rel reticuloendotheliosis viral oncogene homolog	2p13-p12	diffuse large B-cell lymphoma
RPS6KB1	Ribosomal protein S6 kinase, 70kDa, polypeptide 1	17q23.1	breast
SKP2	S-phase kinase-associated protein 2, E3 ubiquitin protein ligase	5p13	lung, esophageal squamous cell carcinoma, soft tissue sarcoma, myxofibrosarcoma
SMURF1	SMAD specific E3 ubiquitin protein ligase 1	7q22.1	pancreas
STARD3	StAR-related lipid transfer (START) domain containing 3	17q11-q12	breast
TSPAN31	Tetraspanin 31	12q14	glioma
WHSC1L1	Wolf-Hirschhorn syndrome candidate 1-like 1	8p11.2	lung
YWHAB	Tyrosine 3-monooxygenase/tryptophan 5-monooxygenase activation protein, beta polypeptide	20q13.1	breast
YWHAQ	Tyrosine 3-monooxygenase/tryptophan 5-monooxygenase activation protein, theta polypeptide	2p25.1	bladder
YWHAZ	Tyrosine 3-monooxygenase/tryptophan 5-monooxygenase activation protein, zeta polypeptide	8q23.1	lung, bladder
ZNF217	Zinc finger protein 217	20q13.2	breast
ZNF639	Zinc finger protein 639	3q26.32	oral squamous cell carcinoma

Detailed Data on Amplified Genes

AKT2

Amplification at 19q13 has been reported in at least 10% high grade serous ovarian carcinoma, but not in low grade disease. Most attention has been directed towards the AKT2 gene at this locus.

AKT2-encoded serine kinase regulates many processes including metabolism, proliferation, cell survival, growth and angiogenesis. siRNA knockdown of AKT2 in an ovarian cancer cell line that contains amplification of this gene resulted in reduced cellular proliferation (Noske et al. 2007).

AR

Several independent studies reported AR gene amplification in approximately 30% of patients with recurrent prostate cancer, and these patients have a 4.569 higher likelihood of responding to a second-line hormonal therapy as compared with patients with no AR amplification (Attar et al. 2009)

ARPC1A and SMURF1

Both may be amplified at 7q22.1 and overexpressed in pancreas cancer. ARPC1A encodes a protein involved in actin polymerization. Its inhibition is associated to a massive reduction in cell migration and invasion (Laurila et al. 2009). The protein encoded by SMURF1 downregulates TGF-β signaling pathway components, such as SMAD4, which is known to be mutated in human pancreatic cancer.

BCL2L2, PAX9, NKX2-1 and NKX2-8

Loci 14q11.2 and 14q13.3 are frequently amplified in lung cancer. At 14q11.2, BCL2L2 is a pro-survivor protein and other genes in this pathway including TP53 are also frequently mutated in lung cancer (Kim et al. 2006). PAX9, NKX2-1, NKX2-8, three genes in the 14q13.3 core region, encode transcription factors with either established lung developmental function (NKX2-1, NKX2-8) or potential lung developmental function (PAX9). It has been suggested that patients with coactivation of NKX2-1 and NKX2-8 pathways could be resistant to standard cisplatin therapy (Hsu et al. 2009)].

CACNA1E

CACNA1E encodes major subunit of the voltage-dependent Ca^{2+} channel Ca(V)2.3. It is amplified in 8% of Wilms tumors and significantly linked to early tumor relapse (Natrajan et al. 2006)

CCND1

11q13 is frequently amplified in various cancers: lung, breast cancer, cervical and oral squamous carcinoma, malignant melanoma, Barrett's adenocarcinoma (Fu et al. 2004). CCND1 encodes cyclin D1, which promotes cell cycle progression through the G1-S phase of the cell cycle (Tashiro et al. 2007)]. CCND1 amplification is generally associated to overexpression and poor prognosis. Inhibition of cyclin D1 expression in a carcinoma cell line, in which CCND1 gene is amplified and overexpressed, was shown to cause reversion of the malignant phenotype.

CCNE1

19q12 is amplified in a subgroup of estrogen receptor-negative high-grade breast cancers. This amplicon comprises nine genes, including cyclin E1 (CCNE1), which has been proposed as its 'driver'. CCNE1-encoded cyclin E1 forms a complex with and functions as a regulatory subunit of cyclin-dependant kinase 2, whose activity is required for cell cycle G1-S transition. CCNE1 silencing was shown to reduce cell viability in cancer cells harboring CCNE1 amplification. These cells were shown to be dependent on CDK2 expression and kinase activity for their survival (Natrajan et al. 2012).

CDK4

Amplification and, in most cases, overexpression of CDK4 was found in breast cancer, glioma, sarcoma and melanoma. CDK4-encoded protein plays a central role in the regulation of the cell cycle G0–G1 transition and is required for the G1-S phase transition. Various selective inhibitors for CDK4 are in development (Shafiq et al. 2012).

CDK6

In approximately 25% of primary myxofibrosarcomas, CDK6 overexpression is mostly driven by gene amplification, associated with adverse prognosticators, and independently predictive of worse outcomes, highlighting its possible causative role in tumor aggressiveness (Tsai et al. 2012). In glioma, knockdown of CDK6 enhances sensitivity to chemotherapy (Li et al. 2012).

CHD1L

1q21 is frequently amplified in hepatocellular carcinoma. It has been implicated in chromatin remodeling and DNA relaxation process required for DNA replication, repair and transcription. CHD1L could contribute to tumor cell migration, invasion, and metastasis by increasing cell motility and inducing filopodia formation and epithelial-mesenchymal transition (Chen et al. 2010).

CKS1B

In breast cancer, oncogene CKS1B amplification is highly correlated to protein overexpression. CKS1B protein (Cks1) binds to the catalytic subunit of the cyclin-dependent kinases and is essential for their biological function. Cks1-depleted breast cancer cells not only exhibit slowed G1 progression, but also accumulate in G2-M due to blocked mitotic entry. Cks1 inhibits apoptosis of cancer cells (Wang et al. 2009a). CKS1B amplification has also been described in multiple myeloma, squamous cell carcinoma and lung cancer, where it is associated to aggressiveness.

COPS3

Amplification at 17q11 is reported to be one of the most common aberrations in osteosarcoma. COPS3 amplification is associated to overexpression (Henriksen et al. 2003). COPS3 encodes a protein targeting p53 to MDM2-mediated ubiquitination and subsequent degradation,

DCUN1D1

Chromosomal amplification at 3q is common to multiple human cancers, but has a specific predilection for squamous cell carcinomas (SCC) of mucosal origin. DCUN1D1 amplification and overexpression in these tumors correlated with poor clinical outcome (Sarkaria et al. 2006).

DYRK2

Its protein product controls cell cycle progression at the G1-S phase. DYRK2 inactivation contributes to cell proliferation and tumor progression. Amplification and overexpression of DYRK2 have been reported in lung and esophageal adenocarcinomas (Miller et al. 2003).

E2F3

Amplification or gain of DNA at 6p22 has been reported in up to a quarter of human bladder cancer. E2F3 occurs within the minimal region of amplification. There is a striking relationship between 6p22 amplification, E2F3 overexpression and lack of Rb expression. The Rb pathway that controls transcription by E2F proteins (including E2F3) has previously been implicated in the development of bladder cancer (Hurst et al. 2008)

EGFR

It encodes epidermal growth factor receptor. EGFR and its three related proteins (the "ERBB family") are receptor tyrosine kinases that play essential roles in both normal physiological conditions and cancerous conditions. In various cancers, EGFR amplification is correlated with high probability to respond to anti-EGFR agents (Giaccone and Wang 2011).

EIF5A2

Amplification of 3q26 is one of the most frequent chromosomal alterations in many solid tumors, including ovarian, lung, esophageal, prostate, breast, and nasopharyngeal cancers. In ovarian cancer, EIF5A2 overexpression was significantly associated with the advanced stage of ovarian cancer. In non-small lung cancer, EIF5A2 overexpression was correlated with local invasion and might serve as an adverse prognostic marker of survival (He et al. 2011). The gene encodes an mRNA-binding protein involved in translation elongation and cell cycle progression.

ERBB2, STARD3 and GRB7

17q13 is frequently amplified breast cancer. Up to 40% of human breast cancers exhibit ERBB2 amplification (up to 25–50 copies) and overexpression, and expression level of the encoded protein was found to be associated with several clinical parameters including overall survival, time to relapse, higher grade and estrogen negativity. Specific therapies targeting ERBB2 breast tumors have been developed, including the use of trastuzumab (Rexer and Arteaga 2012). In breast cancer, the minimal region of amplification at 17q13 included GRB7 and STARD3, in addition to ERBB2. Knockdown of each of the three genes individually results in decreased proliferation, but only in breast cells containing the 17q13 amplicon.

ERBB2 is also amplified in a significant minority of ovarian, gastric, endometrial, esophageal, bladder and lung cancers, as well as in oral and oropharyngeal squamous cell carcinoma and medulloblastoma. In most cases, ERBB2 overexpression is associated with poorer prognosis.

FADD

It encodes an adaptor for relaying apoptotic signals, which also plays an important role in the growth and regulation of the cell cycle. Its amplification and overexpression have been detected in oral squamous cell carcinoma and were significantly correlated with lymph node metastasis and reduced survival (Prapinjumrune et al. 2010).

FGFR1 and WHSC1L1

Amplification at 8p11-12 has been observed in various cancers (including breast, lung, rhabdomyosarcoma…). To date, in breast cancer, the role of FGFR1 as the driver breast cancer oncogene affected in the 8p11-12 amplification is not widely accepted, but its amplification has been reported to be associated with poor prognosis, especially in patients with estrogen-receptor positive tumors (Jang et al. 2012)]. FGFR1 amplification and overexpression have also been reported in rhabdomosarcoma (Missiaglia et al. 2009) and in squamous cell lung cancer (Dutt et al. 2011).

Amplification and over expression of WHSC1L1 were observed in non-small cell lung cancer specimens (Tonon et al. 2005). WHSC1L1 is also involved in a chromosomal translocation in acute myeloid leukemia, t(8;11)(p11.2; p15), that preserves all of the domains in WHSC1L1, excluding one PWWP domain. WHSC1L1 encodes a histone methyltransferase critical in maintaining chromatin integrity.

GATA6

18q11.2 amplification has been found in pancreatobiliary cancer, while it is uncommon in many other tumor types. The smallest shared amplification at 18q11.2 included GATA6, a transcriptional regulator previously linked to normal pancreas development. siRNA mediated knockdown of GATA6 in pancreatic cancer cell lines with amplification led to reduced cell proliferation, cell cycle progression, and colony formation (Kwei et al. 2008).

GPC5

Genomic amplification of the 13q31-32 region is reported in many cancers, including rhabdomyosarcoma. In the minimum overlapping region of amplification at 13q31-32, it has been observed that GPC5 was the only gene consistently expressed and up-regulated in all cases with amplification. In the context of sarcomagenesis, it has been proposed that GPC5 enhances fibroblast growth factor signaling that leads to mesodermal cell proliferation (Williamson et al. 2007).

JUN

It encodes a component (c-Jun) of the AP-1 transcription factor and is consequently involved in a wide range of pivotal cellular processes, including cell proliferation, transformation, and apoptosis. Genomic amplification of c-Jun is observed in aggressive sarcomas and has been implicated as a mechanism of progression from well-differentiated to dedifferentiated liposarcoma, by blocking an early step of adipocyte differentiation (Mariani et al. 2007).

KIT

Testicular germ cell tumors (TGCT) are the leading cause of cancer deaths in young male Caucasians. 4q12 is frequently amplified in these tumors and KIT appears to be the only gene consistently mapping within the amplicon. In keeping with the copy number changes, expression of KIT was significantly greater in seminomas than in non-seminomatous testicular cancers (Goddard et al. 2007).

MAP3K5

Malignant fibrous histiocytomas are aggressive tumors without any definable line of differentiation. In such tumors, MAP3K5 is in the minimal region of amplification at 6q23. The gene encodes a mitogen-activated protein kinase kinase kinase of the JNK-MAPK signaling pathway which could inhibit the adipocytic differentiation process of the tumor cells (Chibon et al. 2004).

MDM2

It encodes a negative regulator of the p53 tumor suppressor. Amplification and /or overexpression of MDM2 occur in many tumors. Increased levels of MDM2 would inactivate the apoptotic and cell cycle arrest functions of p53, as do deletion or mutation of p53, common events in cancer genesis. In a study of 3889 samples from tumors or xenografts from 28 tumor types, the overall frequency of MDM2 amplification was 7%. Gene amplification was observed in 19 tumor types, with the highest frequency observed in soft tissue tumors (20%), osteosarcomas (16%) and esophageal carcinomas (13%). More than 5% of lung, breast and brain tumors were affected (Momand et al. 1998).

MDM4

Its amplification is common in glioblastoma multiforme (Rao et al. 2010) and it directly contributes to tumor formation by inhibiting p53 tumor suppressor activity. Retinoma is a benign variant of retinoblastoma that was initially considered a tumor regression, but recent evidences suggest that it rather represents a pre-malignant lesion issued from normal retina. It has been suggested that MDM4 gain might be involved in the early transition from normal retina to retinoma (Sampieri et al. 2008).

MED29

In a study of 16 pancreatic cancer cell lines and 31 primary tumors, seven genes in the 19q13 amplicon had consistently elevated expression levels. Loss-of-function screen by RNA interference showed that MED29 silencing resulted in G0-G1 cell cycle arrest and increased apoptosis in pancreatic cancer cells (Kuuselo et al. 2007).

MET

It encodes a cell membrane tyrosine kinase receptor for hepatocyte growth factor (HGF). MET conveys mitogenic, motogenic and proangiogenic signals, important during embryonic development and during the development of cancer. Activation of the HGF-MET pathway seems to be associated with a poor prognosis in lung cancer. A number of novel therapeutic agents that target the HGF-MET pathway are in development, including the inhibitor crizotinib (Okamoto et al. 2012)]. In gastric cancers, MET amplification is associated with gene overexpression. Overexpression of MET in the presence of amplification is associated with poorer clinical outcome or more advanced disease.

MITF

It is strongly amplified in 15% to 20% of metastatic melanomas. MITF amplification is associated with a reduced survival in metastatic melanoma patients, and reduction of MITF activity was shown to sensitize melanoma cell lines to chemotherapeutics, suggesting MITF gene copy number as a predictive biomarker of response and survival after chemotherapy (Ugurel et al. 2007)

MTDH

In breast cancer, MTDH amplification and overexpression are associated with poor survival and higher risk of progression (Hu et al. 2009)].

MYC

8q24 is frequently amplified in various cancers and MYC is the gene most extensively examined in this amplicon. The MYC-encoded oncoprotein coordinates a number of normal physiological processes necessary for growth and expansion of somatic cells by controlling the expression of numerous target genes. Deregulation of MYC as a consequence of carcinogenic events enforces cells to undergo a transition to a hyperproliferative state. This increases the risk of additional oncogenic mutations that in turn can result in further tumor progression (Larsson and Henriksson 2010). A significant minority of cancers affecting breast, colon, stomach, prostate, liver, lung, as well as medulloblastoma, malignant melanoma and osteosarcoma, express amplified MYC (Dang 2012). This event is generally associated with poor prognosis.

MYCL1

It is frequently amplified in small cell lung cancer (SCLC), where amplification of other MYC family genes, including MYC and MYCN, may also be observed. These events were associated with shorter survival times (Kim et al. 2006)

MYCN

It belongs to the MYC family of proto-oncogenes and is fundamental in the development of the peripheral and central nervous systems. It has been proposed that it could serve as a specific and selective drug target for peripheral and central nervous system tumors (Pession and Tonelli 2005). In neuroblastoma, MYCN amplification is one of the few prediction markers for adverse outcome.

NCOA3, YWHAB (See Below), ZNF217, and AURKA

These genes at 20q13 are frequently amplified in various cancers. ZNF217 is a transcription factor. It has oncogenic potential since it can immortalize breast epithelial cells and can suppress cell death by acting on the AKT pathway. AURKA encodes a kinase that contributes to the regulation of cell cycle progression. The correlation of AURKA amplification and higher breast cancer grade has been reported. AURKA overexpression induces centrosome amplification and aneuploidy in human breast cells and a correlation between mRNA overexpression and chromosome instability has been reported in breast cancer. NCOA3 is amplified in up to 10% of breast cancers. Amplification is associated with mRNA and protein overexpression, which can be associated with clinical outcome (Bautista et al. 1998).

PAK1

It is amplified in several human cancer types, including 30--33% of breast tumor samples and cancer cell lines. PAK1 encodes a protein that coordinately activates MAPK and MET signaling pathways. Disruption of these activities inhibits PAK1-driven anchorage-independent growth (Shrestha et al. 2012).

PIK3CA

It encodes the p110a catalytic subunit of phosphatidylinositol-3-kinase. It is frequently amplified in ovarian cancer. Amplification of PIK3CA is associated with overexpression. Amplification correlates with resistance to chemotherapy (Kolasa et al. 2009).

PRKCI

Gain of 3q26, including PRKCI, is a common event in squamous cell carcinomas. In these tumors, PRKCI amplification was highly correlated with protein (PKCι) overexpression. Positive correlation was found for PRKCI between amplification and tumor size, lymph node metastasis and clinical stage (Yang et al. 2008). Of note, PKCι expression is elevated in NSCLC tumors and cell lines, and PKCι is required for the transformed phenotype of NSCLC cells harboring oncogenic Kras mutation (Regala et al. 2009)

RAB25

Amplification of at 1q22 is centered on the RAB25 small GTPase, which is implicated in apical vesicle trafficking. It is amplified in approximately half of ovarian and breast cancers and determines aggressiveness (Cheng et al. 2004)

REL

It has been proposed that REL is the critical target gene of 2p12-16 amplification in diffuse large B-cell lymphoma (DLBCL). However, conflicting data suggest that REL may not be the functional target of the amplification event (Houldsworth et al. 2004).

RPS6KB1 and PPM1D

17q22-23 is commonly amplified and has been associated with cancer progression in various cancer types. RPS6KB1 and PPM1D are two genes in this amplicon that are overexpressed in breast cancer and have been shown to contribute to tumor formation and/or progression. RPS6KB1-encoded protein is a ribosomal protein that is involved in the progression from the G1 to S phase of the cell cycle (van der Hage et al. 2004). PPM1D-encoded protein is a p53-induced Serine/Threonine phosphatase that accumulates after DNA damage. It dephosphorylates and inactivates several proteins critical for cellular stress responses. PPM1D amplification and overexpression are almost exclusively found in breast cancer with wild type p53 (Rauta et al. 2006).

SKP2

In esophageal squamous cell carcinoma, SKP2 amplification and overexpression correlated significantly with tumor stage and positive lymph node metastasis. It was shown that elevated expression of SKP2 protected cancer cells from anoikis, and this effect was mediated, at least in part, by the phosphoinositidyl 3-kinase-Akt pathway (Wang et al. 2009b). In small cell lung cancers (SCLC), expression levels of SKP2 protein correlated with the DNA copy-number of the gene (Yokoi et al. 2002).

TSPAN31 (Formerly SAS)

In glioma, TSPAN31 and CDK4 are frequently coamplified and overexpressed. The TSPAN31 gene product belongs to the transmembrane 4 protein superfamily (TM4SF), other members of which have been found to be involved in signal transduction and growth control as well as suppression of metastatic potential. Thus, overexpression of TSPAN31 protein due to gene amplification could result in disturbances of cellular growth control (Reifenberger et al. 1996).

YWHAB, YWHAQ, YWHAZ

These genes encode proteins of the 14-3-3 family. There are seven 14-3-3 isoforms, which are believed to function as general survival factors by enhancing pro-survival signaling and suppressing pro-apoptotic proteins (Heidenblad et al. 2008).

ZNF639

Its amplification was associated with its overexpression in esophageal squamous cell carcinoma and high ZNF639 expression was shown to be an independent indicator of poor survival in this cancer. Ectopic expression of ZNF639 promoted cell growth but knockdown suppressed growth in esophageal cancer cells (Imoto et al. 2003).

References

Attar RM, Takimoto CH, Gottardis MM. Castration-resistant prostate cancer: locking up the molecular escape routes. *Clin Cancer Res.* 2009 May 15;15(10):3251-5.

Bautista S, Vallès H, Walker RL, Anzick S, Zeillinger R, Meltzer P, Theillet C. In breast cancer, amplification of the steroid receptor coactivator gene AIB1 is correlated with estrogen and progesterone receptor positivity. *Clin Cancer Res.* 1998 Dec;4(12):2925-9.

Chen L, Chan TH, Yuan YF, Hu L, Huang J, Ma S, Wang J, Dong SS, Tang KH, Xie D, et al. CHD1L promotes hepatocellular carcinoma progression and metastasis in mice and is associated with these processes in human patients. *J Clin Invest.* 2010 Apr;120(4):1178-91.

Cheng KW, Lahad JP, Kuo WL, Lapuk A, Yamada K, Auersperg N, Liu J, Smith-McCune K, Lu KH, Fishman D, Gray JW, Mills GB. The RAB25 small GTPase determines aggressiveness of ovarian and breast cancers. *Nat Med.* 2004 Nov;10(11):1251-6.

Chibon F, Mariani O, Derré J, Mairal A, Coindre JM, Guillou L, Sastre X, Pédeutour F, Aurias A. ASK1 (MAP3K5) as a potential therapeutic target in malignant fibrous histiocytomas with 12q14-q15 and 6q23 amplifications. *Genes Chromosomes Cancer.* 2004 May;40(1):32-7.

Dang CV. MYC on the path to cancer. *Cell.* 2012 Mar 30;149(1):22-35.

Dutt A, Ramos AH, Hammerman PS, Mermel C, Cho J, Sharifnia T, Chande A, Tanaka KE, Stransky N, Greulich H, et al. Inhibitor-sensitive FGFR1 amplification in human non-small cell lung cancer. *PLoS One.* 2011;6(6):e20351.

Fu M, Wang C, Li Z, Sakamaki T, Pestell RG. Minireview: Cyclin D1: normal and abnormal functions. *Endocrinology.* 2004 Dec;145(12):5439-47.

Giaccone G, Wang Y. Strategies for overcoming resistance to EGFR family tyrosine kinase inhibitors. *Cancer Treat Rev.* 2011 Oct;37(6):456-64.

Goddard NC, McIntyre A, Summersgill B, Gilbert D, Kitazawa S, Shipley J. KIT and RAS signalling pathways in testicular germ cell tumours: new data and a review of the literature. *Int J Androl.* 2007 Aug;30(4):337-48.

He LR, Zhao HY, Li BK, Liu YH, Liu MZ, Guan XY, Bian XW, Zeng YX, Xie D. Overexpression of eIF5A-2 is an adverse prognostic marker of survival in stage I non-small cell lung cancer patients. *Int J Cancer.* 2011 Jul 1;129(1):143-50.

Heidenblad M, Lindgren D, Jonson T, Liedberg F, Veerla S, Chebil G, Gudjonsson S, Borg A, Månsson W, Höglund M. Tiling resolution array CGH and high density expression profiling of urothelial carcinomas delineate genomic amplicons and candidate target genes specific for advanced tumors. *BMC Med Genomics.* 2008 Jan 31;1:3.

Henriksen J, Aagesen TH, Maelandsmo GM, Lothe RA, Myklebost O, Forus A. Amplification and overexpression of COPS3 in osteosarcomas potentially target TP53 for proteasome-mediated degradation. *Oncogene.* 2003 Aug 14;22(34):5358-61.

Houldsworth J, Olshen AB, Cattoretti G, Donnelly GB, Teruya-Feldstein J, Qin J, Palanisamy N, Shen Y, Dyomina K, Petlakh M, et al. Relationship between REL amplification, REL function, and clinical and biologic features in diffuse large B-cell lymphomas. *Blood.* 2004 Mar 1;103(5):1862-8.

Hsu DS, Acharya CR, Balakumaran BS, Riedel RF, Kim MK, Stevenson M, Tuchman S, Mukherjee S, Barry W, Dressman HK, et al. Characterizing the developmental pathways

TTF-1, NKX2-8, and PAX9 in lung cancer. *Proc Natl Acad Sci U S A.* 2009 Mar 31;106(13):5312-7.

Hu G, Chong RA, Yang Q, Wei Y, Blanco MA, Li F, Reiss M, Au JL, Haffty BG, Kang Y. MTDH activation by 8q22 genomic gain promotes chemoresistance and metastasis of poor-prognosis breast cancer. *Cancer Cell.* 2009 Jan 6;15(1):9-20.

Hurst CD, Tomlinson DC, Williams SV, Platt FM, Knowles MA. Inactivation of the Rb pathway and overexpression of both isoforms of E2F3 are obligate events in bladder tumours with 6p22 amplification. *Oncogene.* 2008 Apr 24;27(19):2716-27.

Imoto I, Yuki Y, Sonoda I, Ito T, Shimada Y, Imamura M, Inazawa J. Identification of ZASC1 encoding a Krüppel-like zinc finger protein as a novel target for 3q26 amplification in esophageal squamous cell carcinomas. *Cancer Res.* 2003 Sep 15;63(18):5691-6.

Jang MH, Kim EJ, Choi Y, Lee HE, Kim YJ, Kim JH, Kang E, Kim SW, Kim IA, Park SY. FGFR1 is amplified during the progression of in situ to invasive breast carcinoma. *Breast Cancer Res.* 2012 Aug 3;14(4):R115.

Kim YH, Girard L, Giacomini CP, Wang P, Hernandez-Boussard T, Tibshirani R, Minna JD, Pollack JR. Combined microarray analysis of small cell lung cancer reveals altered apoptotic balance and distinct expression signatures of MYC family gene amplification. *Oncogene.* 2006 Jan 5;25(1):130-8.

Kolasa IK, Rembiszewska A, Felisiak A, Ziolkowska-Seta I, Murawska M, Moes J, Timorek A, Dansonka-Mieszkowska A, Kupryjanczyk J. PIK3CA amplification associates with resistance to chemotherapy in ovarian cancer patients. *Cancer Biol Ther.* 2009 Jan;8(1):21-6.

Kuuselo R, Savinainen K, Azorsa DO, Basu GD, Karhu R, Tuzmen S, Mousses S, Kallioniemi A. Intersex-like (IXL) is a cell survival regulator in pancreatic cancer with 19q13 amplification. *Cancer Res.* 2007 Mar 1;67(5):1943-9.

Kwei KA, Bashyam MD, Kao J, Ratheesh R, Reddy EC, Kim YH, Montgomery K, Giacomini CP, Choi YL, Chatterjee S, et al. Genomic profiling identifies GATA6 as a candidate oncogene amplified in pancreatobiliary cancer. *PLoS Genet.* 2008 May 23;4(5):e1000081.

Larsson LG, Henriksson MA. The Yin and Yang functions of the Myc oncoprotein in cancer development and as targets for therapy. *Exp Cell Res.* 2010 May 1;316(8):1429-37.

Laurila E, Savinainen K, Kuuselo R, Karhu R, Kallioniemi A. Characterization of the 7q21-q22 amplicon identifies ARPC1A, a subunit of the Arp2/3 complex, as a regulator of cell migration and invasion in pancreatic cancer. *Genes Chromosomes Cancer.* 2009 Apr;48(4):330-9.

Li B, He H, Tao BB, Zhao ZY, Hu GH, Luo C, Chen JX, Ding XH, Sheng P, Dong Y, et al. Knockdown of CDK6 enhances glioma sensitivity to chemotherapy. *Oncol Rep.* 2012 Sep;28(3):909-14.

Mariani O, Brennetot C, Coindre JM, Gruel N, Ganem C, Delattre O, Stern MH, Aurias A. JUN oncogene amplification and overexpression block adipocytic differentiation in highly aggressive sarcomas. *Cancer Cell.* 2007 Apr;11(4):361-74.

Miller CT, Aggarwal S, Lin TK, Dagenais SL, Contreras JI, Orringer MB, Glover TW, Beer DG, Lin L. Amplification and overexpression of the dual-specificity tyrosine-(Y)-phosphorylation regulated kinase 2 (DYRK2) gene in esophageal and lung adenocarcinomas. *Cancer Res.* 2003 Jul 15;63(14):4136-43.

Missiaglia E, Selfe J, Hamdi M, Williamson D, Schaaf G, Fang C, Koster J, Summersgill B, Messahel B, Versteeg R, et al. Genomic imbalances in rhabdomyosarcoma cell lines affect expression of genes frequently altered in primary tumors: an approach to identify candidate genes involved in tumor development. *Genes Chromosomes Cancer.* 2009 Jun;48(6):455-67.

Momand J, Jung D, Wilczynski S, Niland J. The MDM2 gene amplification database. *Nucleic Acids Res.* 1998 Aug 1;26(15):3453-9.

Natrajan R, Little SE, Reis-Filho JS, Hing L, Messahel B, Grundy PE, Dome JS, Schneider T, Vujanic GM, Pritchard-Jones K, Jones C. Amplification and overexpression of CACNA1E correlates with relapse in favorable histology Wilms' tumors. *Clin Cancer Res.* 2006 Dec 15;12(24):7284-93.

Natrajan R, Mackay A, Wilkerson PM, Lambros MB, Wetterskog D, Arnedos M, Shiu KK, Geyer FC, Langerød A, Kreike B, et al. Functional characterization of the 19q12 amplicon in grade III breast cancers. *Breast Cancer Res.* 2012 Mar 20;14(2):R53.

Noske A, Kaszubiak A, Weichert W, Sers C, Niesporek S, Koch I, Schaefer B, Sehouli J, Dietel M, Lage H, Denkert C. Specific inhibition of AKT2 by RNA interference results in reduction of ovarian cancer cell proliferation: increased expression of AKT in advanced ovarian cancer. *Cancer Lett.* 2007 Feb 8;246(1-2):190-200.

Okamoto W, Okamoto I, Arao T, Kuwata K, Hatashita E, Yamaguchi H, Sakai K, Yanagihara K, Nishio K, Nakagawa K. Antitumor action of the MET tyrosine kinase inhibitor crizotinib (PF-02341066) in gastric cancer positive for MET amplification. *Mol Cancer Ther.* 2012 Jul;11(7):1557-64.

Pession A, Tonelli R. The MYCN oncogene as a specific and selective drug target for peripheral and central nervous system tumors. *Curr Cancer Drug Targets.* 2005 Jun;5(4):273-83.

Prapinjumrune C, Morita K, Kuribayashi Y, Hanabata Y, Shi Q, Nakajima Y, Inazawa J, Omura K. DNA amplification and expression of FADD in oral squamous cell carcinoma. *J Oral Pathol Med.* 2010 Aug 1;39(7):525-32.

Rao SK, Edwards J, Joshi AD, Siu IM, Riggins GJ. A survey of glioblastoma genomic amplifications and deletions. *J Neurooncol.* 2010 Jan;96(2):169-79.

Rauta J, Alarmo EL, Kauraniemi P, Karhu R, Kuukasjärvi T, Kallioniemi A. The serine-threonine protein phosphatase PPM1D is frequently activated through amplification in aggressive primary breast tumours. *Breast Cancer Res Treat.* 2006 Feb;95(3):257-63.

Regala RP, Davis RK, Kunz A, Khoor A, Leitges M, Fields AP. Atypical protein kinase C{iota} is required for bronchioalveolar stem cell expansion and lung tumorigenesis. *Cancer Res.* 2009 Oct 1;69(19):7603-11.

Reifenberger G, Ichimura K, Reifenberger J, Elkahloun AG, Meltzer PS, Collins VP. Refined mapping of 12q13-q15 amplicons in human malignant gliomas suggests CDK4/SAS and MDM2 as independent amplification targets. *Cancer Res.* 1996 Nov 15;56(22):5141-5.

Rexer BN, Arteaga CL. Intrinsic and acquired resistance to HER2-targeted therapies in HER2 gene-amplified breast cancer: mechanisms and clinical implications. *Crit Rev Oncog.* 2012;17(1):1-16.

Sampieri K, Mencarelli MA, Epistolato MC, Toti P, Lazzi S, Bruttini M, De Francesco S, Longo I, Meloni I, Mari F, et al. Genomic differences between retinoma and retinoblastoma. *Acta Oncol.* 2008;47(8):1483-92.

Sarkaria I, O-charoenrat P, Talbot SG, Reddy PG, Ngai I, Maghami E, Patel KN, Lee B, Yonekawa Y, Dudas M, et al. Squamous cell carcinoma related oncogene/DCUN1D1 is highly conserved and activated by amplification in squamous cell carcinomas. *Cancer Res.* 2006 Oct 1;66(19):9437-44.

Shafiq MI, Steinbrecher T, Schmid R. Fascaplysin as a Specific Inhibitor for CDK4: Insights from Molecular Modelling. *PLoS One.* 2012;7(8):e42612.

Shimizu N. Extrachromosomal double minutes and chromosomal homogeneously staining regions as probes for chromosome research. *Cytogenet Genome Res.* 2009;124(3-4): 312-26.

Shrestha Y, Schafer EJ, Boehm JS, Thomas SR, He F, Du J, Wang S, Barretina J, Weir BA, Zhao JJ, Polyak K, Golub TR, Beroukhim R, Hahn WC. PAK1 is a breast cancer oncogene that coordinately activates MAPK and MET signaling. *Oncogene.* 2012 Jul 19;31(29):3397-408.

Tashiro E, Tsuchiya A, Imoto M. Functions of cyclin D1 as an oncogene and regulation of cyclin D1 expression. *Cancer Sci.* 2007 May;98(5):629-35.

Tonon G, Wong KK, Maulik G, Brennan C, Feng B, Zhang Y, Khatry DB, Protopopov A, You MJ, Aguirre AJ, et al. High-resolution genomic profiles of human lung cancer. *Proc Natl Acad Sci U S A.* 2005 Jul 5;102(27):9625-30.

Tsai JW, Li CF, Kao YC, Wang JW, Fang FM, Wang YH, Wu WR, Wu LC, Hsing CH, Li SH, et al. Recurrent Amplification at 7q21.2 Targets CDK6 Gene in Primary Myxofibrosarcomas and Identifies CDK6 Overexpression as an Independent Adverse Prognosticator. *Ann Surg Oncol.* 2012 Aug;19(8):2716-25.

Ugurel S, Houben R, Schrama D, Voigt H, Zapatka M, Schadendorf D, Bröcker EB, Becker JC. Microphthalmia-associated transcription factor gene amplification in metastatic melanoma is a prognostic marker for patient survival, but not a predictive marker for chemosensitivity and chemotherapy response. *Clin Cancer Res.* 2007 Nov 1;13(21):6344-50.

van der Hage JA, van den Broek LJ, Legrand C, Clahsen PC, Bosch CJ, Robanus-Maandag EC, van de Velde CJ, van de Vijver MJ. Overexpression of P70 S6 kinase protein is associated with increased risk of locoregional recurrence in node-negative premenopausal early breast cancer patients. *Br J Cancer.* 2004 Apr 19;90(8):1543-50.

Wang XC, Tian LL, Tian J, Wu HL, Meng AM. Overexpression of Cks1 is associated with poor survival by inhibiting apoptosis in breast cancer. *J Cancer Res Clin Oncol.* 2009a Oct;135(10):1393-401.

Wang XC, Wu YP, Ye B, Lin DC, Feng YB, Zhang ZQ, Xu X, Han YL, Cai Y, Dong JT, *et al.* Suppression of anoikis by SKP2 amplification and overexpression promotes metastasis of esophageal squamous cell carcinoma. *Mol Cancer Res.* 2009b Jan;7(1):12-22.

Williamson D, Selfe J, Gordon T, Lu YJ, Pritchard-Jones K, Murai K, Jones P, Workman P, Shipley J. Role for amplification and expression of glypican-5 in rhabdomyosarcoma. *Cancer Res.* 2007 Jan 1;67(1):57-65.

Yang YL, Chu JY, Luo ML, Wu YP, Zhang Y, Feng YB, Shi ZZ, Xu X, Han YL, Cai Y, et al. Amplification of PRKCI, located in 3q26, is associated with lymph node metastasis in esophageal squamous cell carcinoma. *Genes Chromosomes Cancer.* 2008 Feb;47(2):127-36.

Yokoi S, Yasui K, Saito-Ohara F, Koshikawa K, Iizasa T, Fujisawa T, Terasaki T, Horii A, Takahashi T, Hirohashi S, Inazawa J. A novel target gene, SKP2, within the 5p13 amplicon that is frequently detected in small cell lung cancers. *Am J Pathol.* 2002 Jul;161(1):207-16.

Chapter 4

Low Penetrance Sites in Cancer: Candidate Genes

Abstract

Advances in high-throughput genotyping technologies have enabled the efficient systematic screening of single-nucleotide polymorphisms (SNPs) throughout the human genome for disease associations in genome-wide association studies (GWAS). In many types of cancer, these studies have identified low penetrance sites, of which some are type-specific while other are more common. However, most of the GWAS-identified SNPs for cancers have small effect sizes and collectively only account for a small fraction of the heritability of cancers.

Introduction

It is well established that many cancer types aggregate in families, with the same type of cancer being 2-5-fold more common in the patient's first-degree relatives than in the general population. These "hereditary" cancers support the existence of a genetic susceptibility for at least some types of tumors. Indeed, various epidemiological, twin and familial aggregation studies have made clear that 20–40% of common tumors such as breast, colorectal, and prostate cancers are inherited. However, the effect of high penetrance tumor susceptibility genes such as BRCA1, BRCA2 (in breast cancer), APC, MSH1, MLH2 and MSH6 (in colorectal cancer) only accounts for a small fraction of these cancers. Recent advances in cancer genetics have led to the identification of novel genes that are relatively rare in the general population, but individually confer moderate risk to cause cancer. For instance, in breast cancer, CHEK2, ATM, BRIP and PALB2, are associated with moderate penetrance.

In the last 5 years, the existence of many low penetrance tumor susceptibility genes has been demonstrated in various cancer types. Such variants are common in the population and, as such, may confer a much higher attributable risk in the general population than rare mutations in high penetrance cancer susceptibility genes. Most of these low-penetrance genes have emerged from genome-wide association studies (GWAS). Contrasting with previous candidate gene association studies (CGAS) focusing on the identification of robustly replicated cancer-associated single nucleotide polymorphisms (SNPs) in particular genes or pathways, GWAS use genotyping platforms that can type hundreds of thousands of SNPs simultaneously. It has been estimated that there are nearly 10 million common SNPs in the human genome. However, because recombination tends to occur at distinct 'hot-spots', neighboring polymorphisms are often strongly correlated (in 'linkage disequilibrium', LD) with each other. The majority of common genetic variants can therefore be evaluated for association using only a few hundred thousands SNPs as tags for all the other variants. Thus, it is possible to conduct GWAS using sets of SNPs that tag most known common variants in the genome, and hence scan for associations without prior knowledge of function or position.

Results from GWAS have been published for the commonest cancers worldwide: breast, prostate, lung, colorectal, melanoma..., each reporting well-validated novel associations. In total, these scans have identified more than 100 new cancer susceptibility loci. Additional scans are ongoing in many other cancer types, including cancers of the hematopoietic system, pancreas, bladder, kidney, testis and ovary.

Genes Associated to Gwas Data

GWAS in Breast Cancer (BC)

In the 1990s, two major susceptibility genes for breast cancer (BC), BRCA1 and BRCA2, were identified. They are associated with greater than a 10-fold increase of BC risk relative to the general population. Other rare and highly penetrant loci were reported in rare hereditary cancer syndromes such as Li-Fraumeni syndrome (gene TP53), Cowden's syndrome (gene PTEN) or Peutz-Jeghers (gene STK11). However, the majority of multiple case BC families do not segregate mutations in these genes. Large case-control association studies were required to identify an intermediate risk group of BC variants—in ATM, BRIP1, CHEK2, PALB2, CASP8 and RAD51C. They generally confer a 2- to 3-fold increased risk of BC. Minor allele frequencies for these variants are typically <0.1%. Nevertheless, after accounting for all the known BC loci, more than 75% of the familial risk of the disease remains unexplained.

In one of the earliest GWAS examining breast tumors in search of low-risk susceptibility sites, robust analysis identified six statistically significant SNPs, all of which were previously unreported for BC. Four of the SNPs were found in regions containing genes: FGFR2, TOX3, MAP3K1 and LSP1 whereas the other two were intergenic SNPs found in 8q24.21 and 5p12 (Easton et al. 2007).

The most strongly associated SNP was rs2981582 in intron 2 of the FGFR2 (fibroblast growth factor receptor 2) gene that is amplified and overexpressed in 5-10% of BC (Fanale et al. 2012). FGFR2 is a receptor tyrosine kinase which may increase proliferation, differentiation and enhance the invasiveness of BC cells. The statistical association between rs2981582 and various other SNPs in intron 2 of FGFR2 and BC has been confirmed by a number of studies. Intron 2 includes highly conserved regions and is dense in transcription factor binding sites that may cooperate in increasing gene expression. rs2981582 was significantly associated with positive estrogen receptor (ER) and progesterone receptor (PgR) status (Garcia-Closas et al. 2008; Riaz et al. 2012).

Table 1. Variant SNPs associated with breast cancer and located in or near specific genes

Gene	Variant SNP	Locus
CASP8	rs17468277	2q33
CDKN2A/B	rs1011970	9p21.3
COX11	rs6504950	17q23
RNF146	rs2180341	6q22.33
ERBB4	rs13393577	2q34
ESR1	rs3734805 rs9383938 rs2046210 rs12662670 rs9397435	6q25.1
FGFR2	rs2981582 rs10736303 rs2981578 rs2981579	10q26.13
H19	rs2107425	11p15.5
LSP1	rs3817198	11p15.5
MAP3K1	rs889312	5q11.2
MRPS30	rs7716600	5q12
NOTCH2	rs11249433	1p11.2
RAD51L1	rs999737 rs10483813 rs3784099	14q24.1
ROPN1L	rs1092913	5p15.2
SLC4A7	rs4973768	3p24
Gene	Variant SNP	Locus
TERT – CLPTM1L locus	rs2736109 rs2736108	5p15.33
TGFB1	rs1982073	19q13.1
TOX3	rs3803662 rs4784227	16q12.1
ZMIZ1	rs704010	10q22.3
ZNF365	rs16917302 rs10995190	10q21.2

The rs3803662 SNP near TOX3 (TOX high mobility group box family member 3, previously known as TNRC9) gene is another SNP with a strong association with BC, in particular, this polymorphism appears to be correlated with bone metastases and estrogen receptor positivity (Campa et al. 2011; Fanale et al. 2012). Of interest, TOX3 expression has been previously associated with the presence of bone metastases derived from breast tumors (Smid et al. 2006). TOX3 is involved in mediating calcium-dependent transcription. The strong association between this locus and BC has been independently confirmed by subsequent GWAS.

The associations between SNPs rs889312 in MAP3K1 and rs3817198 in LSP1 and BC are now well established. Mitogen-activated protein kinase 3 K1 is part of the MAPK cell signaling pathway implicated in cellular response to mitogens. LSP1 encodes lymphocyte-specific protein 1, an F-actin-bundling cytoskeletal protein that is expressed in hematopoietic and endothelial cells. LSP1 has been implicated in malignant lymphoma and Hodgkin's disease (Marafioti et al. 2003), and other variants in this gene have been associated with the risk of developing non-Hodgkin's lymphoma. No relationship between MAP3K1 or LSP1 expression and BC was demonstrated before the introduction of GWAS studies.

Other confirmed associations with BC have been found for SNPs in or near ESR1 (estrogen receptor alpha), RAD51L1 (DNA repair protein RAD51 homolog 2), CASP8 (caspase 8), TGFB1 (transforming growth factor beta 1), COX11 (COX11 cytochrome c oxidase assembly homolog (yeast)), ZNF365 (zinc finger protein 365) and SLC4A7 (solute carrier family 4, sodium bicarbonate cotransporter, member 7). The product of RAD51L1 is known to interact with RAD51, which is a breast and ovarian cancer susceptibility gene.

In view of the importance of estrogens in a majority of BC, the association between SNPs in ESR1 and BC is particularly interesting. An association between rs2046210 and BC susceptibility was originally discovered and confirmed in a Chinese population. It was later identified in Japanese and in European populations. An association involving SNP rs12662670 was first identified in Europeans. A recent study showed that these two SNPs were independently associated with BC risk in Asians and in Europeans. Of them, the one tagged by rs2046210 was associated with a greater risk of ER-negative tumors (Hein et al. 2012).

Six single-nucleotide polymorphisms, including rs2046210 (ESR1), rs12662670 (ESR1), rs3803662 (TOX3), rs999737 (RAD51L1), rs8170 (19p13.1), and rs8100241 (19p13.1) were significantly associated with the risk of triple-negative BC (Stevens et al. 2011). Another study identified rs3803662 (TOX3), rs889312 (MAP3K1), rs3817198 (LSP1) and rs13387042 (2q35); however, only two rs3803662 (TOX3) and rs13387042 were associated with tumors with the core basal phenotype (Broeks et al. 2011).

Variants in ZNF365 (rs10995190), LSP1 (rs3817198) and RAD51L1 (rs10483813) have been associated to mammographic density (Lindström et al. 2011; Vachon et al. 2012). Among premenopausal women, rs3817198 (LSP1) and rs12443621, near TOX3, were marginally associated with mammographic density (Tamimi et al. 2008).

GWAS in Prostate Cancer (PC)

Prostate cancer (PC) demonstrates strong familial clustering but high penetrance genes have yet to be identified and replicated. The most likely candidate so far is BRCA2, which is associated with a 20-fold increased risk relative to the general population. GWAS studies have been fruitful in identifying many replicated variants, all with OR <2 and most with OR <1.3. Nevertheless, the cumulative effects of these loci explain at least 20% of the familial risk.

Many of these variants are in intergenic regions at 3p12, 3q21, 8q24, 11q13, 17q24, 19q13 and 22q13.2. However, other variants are in or near genes such as CTBP2 (C-terminal binding protein 2), CTDSPL (CTD (carboxy-terminal domain, RNA polymerase II, polypeptide A) small phosphatase-like), EHBP1 (EH domain binding protein 1), EPAS1 (endothelial PAS domain-containing protein 1, formerly HIF2A), IGF1/IGF2 (insulin-like growth factor 1/ insulin-like growth factor 1 - 11p15), ITGA6 (integrin alpha 6), JAZF1 (JAZF zinc finger 1), KLK3 (kallikrein-related peptidase 3), LMTK2 (lemur tyrosine kinase 2), MSMB (microseminoprotein beta), NKX3.1 (NK3 homeobox 1), NUDT10/NUDT11 (nudix (nucleoside diphosphate linked moiety X)-type motif 10/11), PDLIM5 (PDZ and LIM domain 5), SLC22A3 (solute carrier family 22 (extraneuronal monoamine transporter), member 3), HNF1B (HNF homeobox 1 beta). Interestingly, several of these variants localize to distinct linkage disequilibrium blocks on 8q24 (see below) (Hindorff et al. 2011).

Table 2. Variant SNPs associated with prostate cancer and located in or near specific genes

Gene	Variant SNP	Locus
CTDSPL	rs9311171	3p22.2
DAB2IP	rs7042542	9q33
	rs1571801	
EHBP1	rs721048	2p15
EPAS1	rs4953347	2p21
FOXP4	rs1983891	6p21.1
GPRC6A, RFX6	rs339331	6p22
HNF1B	rs11868513	17q12
	rs4430796	
	rs7501939	
	rs11649743	
Gene	Variant SNP	Locus
IGF2, IGF2A, INS, TH	rs7127900	11p15
ITGA6	rs12621278	2q31
JAZF1	rs10486567	7p15
	rs6968704	
KLK3	rs2735839	19q13.33
	rs17632542	
LMTK2	rs6465657	7q21.3
MSMB	rs10993994	10q11.23
NKX3.1	rs1512268	8p21
NUDT10/11	rs5945572	Xp11.22
	rs5945619	
PDLIM5	rs17021918	4q22
	rs12500426	
SLC22A3	rs9364554	6q25.3
SRRM1L	rs13254738	8q24.21
TCF2	rs4430796	17q12
	rs7501939	
TERT	rs2242652	5p15.33
TET2	rs7679673	4q24
TNRC6B	rs12628051	22q13.1

CTBP2 may associate to chromatin-modifying complexes, which link cellular metabolism to gene transcription. It plays a role in the maintenance of mitotic fidelity (Birts et al. 2011). It could establish a pattern of gene expression that favors pluripotency and asymmetric self-renewal in embryonal stem cells (Tarleton et al. 2010). CTDSPL is hypermutated in various cancers, supporting a role of tumor suppressor gene (TSG); its product could collaborate with that of the TSG RASSF1A (RAS association domain family 1A) in cell cycle arrest (Kashuba et al. 2009). Of note, in PC, RASSF1A gene silencing is observed in over 70% of cases (Amin and Banerjee 2012). EPAS1 belongs to a family of hypoxia-inducible factors that promote key carcinogenic processes such as angiogenesis and metastasis. Under hypoxic conditions, which are common in malignant tumors, EPAS1 directly binds and activates the transcription factor POU5F1, which may lead to tumorigenesis (Ciampa et al. 2011). Various SNPs in both JAZF1 and HNF1B have been associated with decreased risk of PC. JAZF1 encodes a transcriptional repressor. In endometrial (but not prostate) cancer, JAZF1 is frequently fused to SUZ12 to produce a protein with anti-apoptotic activity. KLK3 encodes prostate-specific antigen (PSA). PSA is widely used as a biomarker for PC detection and disease monitoring. Variants rs2735839 and rs17632542 have been shown to be associated with PSA levels and rs17632542 is a non-synonymous coding SNP (Ile179Thr) in KLK3 (Kote-Jarai et al. 2011). MSMB is an immunoglobulin superfamily protein synthesized by prostate epithelial cells and secreted into seminal plasma. The rs10993994 variant, which is located in the MSMB promoter, has been associated with the risk of PC in several independent GWAS; its ability to reduce promoter activity suggests that it could lower MSMB in benign tissue leading to increased prostate cancer risk (Whitaker et al. 2010). Tumor suppressor gene NKX3-1 encodes a prostate specific homeobox gene. It plays an important role in normal differentiation of the prostatic epithelium while its loss of function is an initiating event in prostate carcinogenesis. It has been suggested that NKX3.1 downregulates IGF-1R expression and inhibits IGF-1R-mediated mitogen-activated protein kinase (MAPK)/ERK and AKT signaling pathways, which might partially leads to the inhibition of IGF-1-induced cell growth (Zhang et al. 2012). NUDT10 and NUDT11 are diphosphoinositol polyphosphate phosphohydrolases that were not previously associated to any cancer. SLC22A3 is known to be markedly underexpressed in aggressive prostate cancers (Chen et al. 2012).

GWAS in Colorectal Cancer (CRC)

As in breast cancer, several key loci in colorectal cancer were discovered in familial or syndromic cases. They include APC and mismatch repair genes MLH1, MSH2, MSH6 and PMS2. Together, these loci account for ~20% of the genetic predisposition to colorectal cancer. A handful of low to moderate penetrance variants have been identified in candidate gene association studies and GWAS: they are in or near BMP2, BMP4, CCND1, CDH1, CDKN1A, EIF3H, GREM1, MTHFR (C677T), POLD3, RHPN2, SHROOM2, SMAD7, TGFBR1, 8q24, 10p14, 11q23.1 and 20p12.3 and are associated with small increases in relative risk and which cumulatively account for ~6% of the excess familial risk (Hindorff et al. 2011).

BMP2 and BMP4 are part of the TGF-β-signaling pathway and are involved in the etiology of colon and rectal cancer (Slattery et al. 2012). GREM1 is antagonist of the bone morphogenetic protein (BMP) pathway activity and a duplication in region upstream of the GREM1 locus is involved in "hereditary mixed polyposis syndrome" (HMPS), characterized by multiple types of colorectal polyp, with colorectal carcinoma occurring in a high proportion of affected individuals (Jaeger et al. 2012). TGFBR1 is seen as the central propagator of TGF-β signaling pathway and a potent modifier of colorectal cancer risk in mice and humans. SMAD7 is another actor in the TGF-β signaling by exerting negative feedback loops on this pathway. These findings strongly suggest that germline variants of the TGF-β superfamily may account for a sizeable proportion of colorectal cancer cases (Bellam and Pasche 2010). This is further supported by the fact that mutations in the TGF-β type II receptor (TGFBR2) are estimated to occur in approximately 30% of colorectal carcinomas and mutations in SMAD4 and BMPR1A are found in patients with familial juvenile polyposis, an autosomal dominant condition associated with an increased risk of colorectal cancer (Bellam and Pasche 2010)

Table 3. Variant SNPs associated with colorectal cancer and located in or near specific genes

Gene	Variant SNP	Locus
BMP2	rs4813802	20p12.3
BMP4	rs4444235	14q22.2
CCND1	rs603965	11q13.3
CDH1	rs9929218	16q22.1
	rs16260	
CDKN1A	rs1321311	6p21
EIF3H	rs16892766	8q23.3
GREM1	rs4779584	15q13
MTHFR	rs1801133	1p36.22
POU5FIP1, HsG57825, DQ515897	rs7014346	8q24.21
POLD3	rs3824999	11q13.4
RHPN2	rs10411210	19q13.11
SHROOM2	rs5934683	Xp22.2
SMAD7	rs4939827	18q21.1
	rs4464148	
TGFBR1	rs7034462	9q22
	rs1156875	

CDH1 encodes E-cadherin, which is involved in invasion and metastasis of cancer cells. It has been shown that CDH1 -C160A polymorphism (rs16260) provides a possible protection against CRC. It has been observed that when EIF3H is overexpressed in normal primary prostate cells, the cells exhibit more rapid proliferation and increased clonogenicity. Furthermore, these cells continue to proliferate at subconfluent densities, well beyond the 36 doublings associated with the senescence of non-overexpressing cells (Zhang et al. 2008). G870A, a variant of cyclin D1 (CCND1) and C677T, a variant of MTHFR, have been identified by candidate gene association studies (Yang et al. 2012; Zhang et al. 2012).

GWAS in Lung Cancer (LC)

Table 4. Variant SNPs associated with lung cancer and located in or near specific genes

Gene	Variant SNP	Locus
AGPHD1	rs8034191	15q25.1
AJAP1-NPHP4	rs9439519	1p36.32
BAT3	rs3117582	6p21.33
CHRNA3	rs6495309	15q25.1
	rs1051730	

Table 4. (Continued)

Gene	Variant SNP	Locus
CHRNA5	rs16969968	15q25.1
CHRNB4	rs7178270	15q25.1
CYP24A1	rs4809957	20q13.2
PSMA4	rs7168796	15q25.1
	rs7164594	
TERT – CLPTM1L locus	rs2736100	5p15.33
	rs401681	
	rs402710	
	rs31489	
	rs2853677	
GPC5	rs2352028	13q31.3
IL3-CSF2-P4HA2	rs247008	5q31.1
IREB2	rs2036534	15q25.1
PPP2R2B-STK32A-DPYSL3	rs2895680	5q32
TP63	rs10937405	3q28
TRNAA-UGC	rs4324798	6p22.1

The etiology of lung cancer (LC) is recognized to be strongly environmental, although there is increasing evidence that genetic factors may also play a role. Family and linkage studies have identified high-penetrance variants in TP53, RB1 and at 6q23–25. More recently, GWAS have consistently identified three loci at genome-wide significance - variants at 5p15.33 (TERT-CLPTM1L), 6p21-6p22.1 (BAG6 (formerly BAT3), TRNAA-UGC) and 15q25.1 (CHRNA3, CHRNA4 and CHRNA5, AGPHD1, IREB2, PSMA4), which explain about 7% of the familial risk of LC. Interestingly, 15q25.1 variants are also associated with chronic obstructive pulmonary disease (COPD) and smoking behavior, a risk factor for LC. Part of the association of 15q25.1 variants with lung cancer can probably be explained by associations with smoking behavior; however, not all studies agree whether they have some degree of independent effects (Hindorff et al. 2011). SNPs associated with LC have also been identified in or near AJAP1-NPHP4, CYP24A1, GPC5, PPP2R2B-STK32A-DPYSL3 and TP63. The product of BAG6, BCL2-associated athanogene 6, is a chaperone that plays a key role in various processes such as apoptosis and regulation of chromatin. CHRNA3, CHRNA4 and CHRNA5 are nicotinic receptor genes. Of note, variant rs16969968 is a nonsynonymous SNP in CHRNA5 leading to an amino acid change (D398N) at a highly conserved site across species in the encoded protein. This finding is notable as it is rare for a GWAS to directly detect potential functionally importance variants. IREB2 is an iron regulatory protein. Interestingly, IREB1, also known as ACO1 and located at 9p21.1, is another iron regulatory protein in which variants have been associated to cancer (melanoma) (see below). PSMA4 (proteasome (prosome, macropain) subunit, alpha type, 4) has been proposed as a strong candidate mediator of LC cell growth, and may directly affect LC susceptibility through its modulation of cell proliferation and apoptosis (Liu et al. 2009). NPHP4, a cilia-associated protein, negatively regulates the Hippo pathway, which has an essential role in tumor suppression and the control of cell proliferation (Habbig et al. 2011). It has been hypothesized that GPC5, a member of glypican family, regulates lung cancer development through a complex pathway network, particularly through Wnt, Hh, and FGF signaling pathways and their interactions (Li et al. 2010). DPYSL3 has been associated with a good interferon-γ response of lung cancer patients undergoing α-galactosylceramide-pulsed dendritic cell therapy (Okita et al. 2010).

TP63 amplification and over-representation are highly associated with the diagnosis of lung cancer. Its product, p63, seen as an 'epithelial organizer', directly impinges on epidermal mesenchymal transition, stemness, senescence, cell death and cell cycle arrest, all determinant in cancer, and thus p63 affects chemosensitivity and chemoresistance (Melino 2011).

GWAS in Upper Aerodigestive and Esophageal Cancers

Table 5. Variant SNPs associated with upper aerodigestive/esophageal cancers and located in or near specific genes

Cancer type	Gene	Variant SNP	Locus
Esophageal cancer	ADH1B	rs1229984	4q23
	ADH1C	rs698 rs1693482	4q23
	ALDH2	rs671 rs886205	12q24.12
	PLCE1	rs2274223	10q23
Upper aerodigestive tract cancers	ADH1B	rs1229984	4q23
	ADH1C	rs698 rs1693482	4q23
	ADH4	rs4148887 rs3805322	4q23
	ADH7	rs1573496 rs284787 rs1154460 rs3737482	4q23
	ALDH2	rs671	12q24.12
	HELQ (formerly HEL308), FAM175A	rs1494961	4q21.23

To date, GWAS have identified susceptibility sites in or near ADH1B (alcohol dehydrogenase 1B), ADH1C (alcohol dehydrogenase 1C), ADH4 (alcohol dehydrogenase 4), ADH7 (alcohol dehydrogenase 7), ALDH2 (aldehyde dehydrogenase 2 family (mitochondrial)), HELQ (helicase, POLQ-like, formerly known as HEL308), FAM175A (family with sequence similarity 175, member A), PLCE1 (phospholipase C epsilon 1).

Most of upper aerodigestive/esophageal cancers are strongly associated with environmental and life style risk factors such as smoking and alcohol. It may therefore be unsurprising that such cancers are associated with polymorphisms in genes encoding enzymes (ADH1B, ADH1C, ADH4, ADH7, and ALDH2) involved in alcohol metabolism.

The products of HELQ and FAM175A are involved in DNA repair. HELQ encodes an helicase; another helicase, named "regulator of telomere elongation helicase 1", is encoded by RTEL1 gene, in which two SNPs have been associated to susceptibility to glioma. Other molecules with helicase activity, such as those encoded by RECQL4, WRN and BLM, are known to be altered in cancer-prone diseases Rothmund–Thomson, Werner and Bloom syndromes, respectively, supporting a major role of helicase activity failure in cancer genesis and/or development. FAM175A encodes a BRCA1-binding partner that mediates BRCA1 function in response to DNA damage (Liu et al. 2007). The rs2274223 SNP in PLCE1 gene, also associated with gastric cancer, encodes a phospholipase that has been shown to play a crucial role in chemical carcinogen-induced skin tumor development (Bai et al. 2004). Phospholipase C epsilon plays a suppressive role in incidence of colorectal cancer and is down-regulated in this cancer type (Wang et al. 2008).

GWAS in Bladder Cancer

Table 6. Variant SNPs associated with bladder cancer and located in or near specific genes

Gene	Variant SNP	Locus
CCNE1	rs8102137	19q12
MYC	rs9624880	8q24.21 (region 6)
NAT2	rs1041983 rs1801280 rs1495741	8p22
PSCA	rs2294008 rs2978974	8q24.21 (region 8)
SLC14A1	rs7238033 rs17674580	18q12.3
TERT- CLPTM1L	rs2736100	5p15.33
TACC3 (near FGFR3)	rs798766	4p16
TP63	rs710521	3q28
UGT1A	rs11892031	2q37.1

In bladder cancer, all known SNPs that have been validated in sufficiently large populations are associated with odds ratios smaller than 1.5. These SNPs are located next to the following genes: MYC, TP63 (tumor protein p63), PSCA (prostate stem cell antigen), the TERT-CLPTM1L locus, FGFR3 (fibroblast growth factor receptor 3), TACC3 (transforming acidic coiled coil 3), NAT2 (arylamine N-acetyltransferases 2), CBX6 (chromobox homolog 6), CCNE1 (cyclin E1), and UGT1A (UDP-glucuronosyltransferase 1A).

TP63 encodes p63, which regulates the expression of FGFR3. p63 is downregulated in muscle-invasive bladder cancers, where it is associated with a worse outcome (Choi et al. 2012).

PSCA encodes a glycosylphosphatidylinositol (GPI)-anchored cell surface protein. Two SNPs in the PSCA gene have been associated with the risk of bladder and gastric cancers. The rs2294008 SNP is a missense SNP that alter the start codon of PSCA. The risk allele has been shown to reduce the transcriptional activity of the PSCA promoter in both gastric and bladder cell lines. This and other observations suggest that PSCA may act as a tumor suppressor. No cases of somatic or germline mutations in the PSCA gene have been reported in any cancers to date (Saeki et al. 2010).

A number of studies support a link between mutations in FGFR3 and bladder cancer, notably tumors of low grade and stage (Kamat and Mathew 2011).

The protein product of TACC3 is a non-motor microtubule-associated protein that is important for mitotic spindle stability and organization.

CBX6 encodes a member of the Polycomb group 1 (PcG1), a complex which maintain transcriptional repression of hundreds of genes involved in development, signaling or cancer using chromatin-based epigenetic mechanisms. A role of CBX6 in cancer has not been documented to date.

The product of NAT2 plays a key role in the metabolism of drugs and environmental chemicals and in the metabolic activation and detoxification of procarcinogens (Agúndez 2008).

CCNE1 locus is frequently amplified in various cancers (Koboldt et al. 2012).

UGT1A encodes a protein allowing the glucuronidation of various targets. UGT1A variants influence the metabolic effects of xenobiotic exposure and therefore have been linked to cancer risk (Strassburg et al. 2008).

GWAS in Other Cancer Types

Cancer type	Gene	Variant SNP	Locus
Acute lymphoblastic leukemia	ARID5B	rs10821936 rs10994982	10q21.2
	CDKN2A	rs3731217	9p21.3
	CEBPE	rs2239633	14q11.2
	IKZF1	rs11978267 rs4132601	7p12.2
Basal cell carcinoma	CDKN2A/B	rs2151280	9p21
	EXOC2	rs12210050	6p25
	KRT5	rs11170164	12q12-13
	MC1R	rs1805007	16q24.3
	PADI4, PADI6, RCC2, ARHGEF10L	rs7538876	1p36.13
	RHOU	rs801114	1q42.13
	TP53	rs78378222 rs12951053	17p13.1
	UBAC2	rs7335046	13q32
Chronic lymphocytic leukemia	GRAMD1B	rs735665	11q24.1
	HLA-DQA1	rs9272219 rs9272535	6p21.32
	HLA-DRB5	rs615672 rs674313 rs502771	6p21.32
	IRF4	rs9378805 rs872071	6p25.3
	IRF8	rs305077 rs391525 rs2292982 rs2292980	16q24.1
	PRKD2	rs11083846	19q13.32
	SP140	rs13397985	2q37.1

(Continued)

Cancer type	Gene	Variant SNP	Locus
Endometrial cancer	HNF1B	rs4430796 rs7501939	17q12
Follicular lymphoma	HLA-DQB1	rs6457327	6p21.3
Gallbladder cancer	DCC	rs7504990	18q21.2
Gastric cancer	MUC1	rs4072037	1q22
	PLCE1	rs2274223	10q23
	PSCA	rs2294008 rs2976392	8q24.21 (region 8)
Glioma	CCDC26	rs4295627 rs891835	8q24.21 (region 7)
	CDKN2A/B	rs4977756 rs1412829	9p21.3
	EGFR	rs730437 rs1468727	7p11.2
	PHLDB1	rs498872	11q23.3
	RTEL1	rs6010620 rs4809324	20q13.33
	TERT, CLPTM1L	rs2736100 rs2853677	5p15.33
Hepatocellular carcinoma	GRIK1	rs455804	21q21.3
	HLA-DQ	rs9272105	6p21.32
	HLA-DR	rs9272105	6p21.32
	MICA	rs2596542	6p21.3
Hodgkins lymphoma	GATA3	rs501764	10p14
	HLA-DRA	rs6903608	6p21.32
	PVT1	rs2019960	8q24.21
	REL	rs1432295	2p16.1
Melanoma	ACO1	rs7855483 rs17288067 rs10813813	9p21.1
	ARNT, SETDB1, LASS2, ANXA9	rs7412746	1q21.3
	ASIP (120 kb upstream)	rs4911414 rs1015362	20q11
	CASP8	rs13016963	2q33
	CDC91L1	rs910873	20q11.22
	CDKN2A/B	rs11552822	9p21.3
	MC1R	rs4785763 rs258322	16q24.3
	NCOA6	rs4911442 rs910871	20q11
	PLA2G6	rs2284063	22q13.1
	SLC45A2	rs35414	
	TERT	rs2853676 rs2242652	5p15.33
	TERT-CLPTM1L	rs401681	5p15.33
	TERF1	rs2981096	8q21.11

Cancer type	Gene	Variant SNP	Locus
	TYR	rs1393350	11q14.3
Multiple myeloma	ULK4	rs1052501	3p22.1
Myeloproliferative neoplasms	JAK2	rs4495487	9p24.1
Nasopharyngeal carcinoma	CDNK2A/B	rs1412829	9p21.3
	GABBR1	rs29232	6p22.1
	HCG9	rs3869062	6p21.33
	HLA-A	rs2517713	6p21.33
	HLA-F	rs3129055	6p22.1
	ITGA9	rs2212020	3p22.2
	MDS1-EVI1	rs6774494	3q26
	TNFRSF19	rs9510787	13q12
Neuroblastoma	BARD1	rs6435862	2q35
	LMO1	rs110419	11p15.4
Ovarian cancer	BNC2	rs10756819 rs12379183 rs3814113 rs7861573	9p22
	BABAM1 (formerly MERIT40)	rs8170	19p13.11
	MYC	rs1516982 rs10098821	8q24
	TERT	rs7726159	5p15.33
Pancreatic cancer	ABO	rs505922	9q34
	TERT - CLPTM1L	rs401681	5p15.33
	NR5A2	rs3790844	1q32.1
Renal cell carcinoma	EPAS1	rs11894252 rs7579899	2p21
	SCARB1	rs4765623	12q24.31
Testicular cancer	DMRT1	rs755383	9p24.3
	KITLG	rs995030 rs1508595	12q21.32
	ATF7IP	rs2900333	12p13.1
	SPRY4	rs4624820	5q31.3
	TERT- CLPTM1L	rs4635969	5p15.33
	BAK1	rs210138	6p21.31
Thyroid cancer	FOXE1	rs965513	9q22.33
	NKX2-1	rs944289	14q13.3
Wilms tumor	DDX1	rs3755132	2p24
	DLG2	rs790356	11q14

About TERT and CLPTM1L (5p15.33)

GWAS have provided evidence that polymorphisms in a region (5p15.33) containing TERT (telomerase reverse transcriptase) and CLPTM1L (cleft lip and palate transmembrane protein 1-like protein) genes are associated with cancer development (Rafnar et al. 2009). That genetic variability in this genomic region can modulate cancer susceptibility was supported by a recent meta-analysis 85 studies enrolling 490, 901 subjects (Mocellin et al.

2012). It is known that mutations in the coding regions of TERT can affect telomerase activity and telomere length, and can create severe clinical phenotypes, including a substantive increase in cancer frequency (Baird 2010). GWAS data further suggest a role of telomere length in controlling underlying cancer risk.

Although a connection of CLPTM1L to cancer is suggested by GWAS, the function of CLPTM1L and its role in tumorigenesis is thus far unknown. CLPTM1L was identified as an up-regulated transcript in a cisplatin resistant ovarian tumor cell line (Yamamoto et al. 2001). A functional role in genotoxic stress induced apoptosis, at least in lung cancer, has been proposed (James et al. 2012).

It is plausible that both TERT and CLPTM1L contribute to susceptibility at 5p15.33, having a co-founder effect.

About CDNK2A, CDNK2B, MTAP, ANRIL (9p21)

Chromosome 9p21 has been implicated in the pathogenesis of various cancers, including acute lymphoblastic leukemia, basal cell carcinoma, breast, cutaneous melanoma, glioma, nasopharyngeal carcinoma. This region includes CDKN2A and CDKN2B (CDKN2A/B, cyclin-dependent kinase inhibitor 2A/B), miR-31, antisense noncoding RNA in the INK4 locus (ANRIL), a GWAS hotspot for multiple phenotypes including cancers, MTAP (methylthioadenosine phosphorylase), a gene with tumor suppressor function.

The CDKN2A/B locus encodes three cell cycle inhibitory, tumor suppressor proteins: p15INK4b encoded by CDKN2B, p16INK4a encoded by CDKN2A and p14ARF encoded by an alternative reading frame of CDKN2A. CDKN2A is one of the most frequently mutated genes in tumors. Somatic deletions and/or mutations of various types have been observed in tumors of the following tissues (among others): genital tract, pleura, pancreas, biliary tract, skin, upper aerodigestive tract, CNS, oesophagus, urinary tract...Among skin tumors, CDKN2A alterations are highly associated with cutaneous melanoma. p15Ink4b is a critical tumor suppressor in the absence of p16Ink4a. This provides an explanation for the frequent loss of the complete CDKN2b-CDKN2a locus in human tumors (Krimpenfort et al. 2007).

Many solid tumors and hematologic malignancies lack expression of the enzyme methylthioadenosine phosphorylase (MTAP), due either to deletion of the MTAP gene or to methylation of the MTAP promoter. MTAP encodes an enzyme that plays a major role in polyamine metabolism and is important for the salvage of both adenine and methionine.

Of peculiar interest is miR-31, as the importance of microRNAs in various diseases has been evidenced only recently. The pleiotropic miR-31 is able to inhibit multiple steps in the metastatic process. miR-31 has also been shown to modulate tumor sensitivity to radiation, by regulating the expression of DNA repair genes (Lynam-Lennon et al. 2012).

The long non-coding RNA ANRIL may block the activity of tumor suppressor genes. ANRIL interacts with SUZ12 (suppressor of zeste 12 homolog), a subunit of the polycomb repression complex 2 (PRC2) and recruits this chromatin-remodelling complex to repress the expression of the tumor suppressor CDKN2B. Moreover, the depletion of ANRIL increases the expression of CDKN2B and inhibits cellular proliferation (Gutschner and Diederichs 2012).

About 8q24 and MYC

First GWAS identified multiple SNPs at the 8q24 locus as strongly associated with prostate cancer. In fact, comprehensive genotyping has identified at least five distinct prostate cancer susceptibility regions within 8q24. Some of these regions are also associated to breast, colorectal, ovarian or bladder cancers, as well as to glioma and chronic lymphocytic leukemia (Varghese and Easton 2010). This pleiotropic effect of 8q24 is rather surprising as this region appears as a "gene desert" (Huppi et al. 2012). However, the role of SNPs located in this desert is increasingly investigated. For instance, SNP rs6983267, associated to colorectal and prostate cancer risk is located 300 kb apart from MYC. Later studies have provided insights that the region harboring the particular risk allele is a transcriptional enhancer that interacts with the MYC. It has recently been observed that the presence of the minor allele of rs6983267 worsened the prognosis of colorectal cancer through up-regulation of MYC transcription (Takatsuno 2012).

At 8q24, MYC is one of the most studied oncogenes stemming from its association with a large number of diseases. It may thus appear as the most likely candidate gene target. However, establishing a functional correlation between SNPs and MYC expression has been surprisingly inconsistent. For instance, SNPs both upstream and downstream of MYC have been linked to ovarian cancer, suggesting MYC is the target gene in this case (Goode EL et al. 2010). However, studies of risk-associated alleles in ovarian cancer have failed to show correlation with MYC expression (Huppi et al. 2012).

Besides MYC, other candidates at 8q24 are PVT1, FAM84B, POU5F1B and PRNC1, but also miRNAs (Huppi et al. 2012)

Conclusion

Cancer genetics has advanced prominently over the past few years in the GWAS era. More than 100 SNPs have been identified. However, these SNPs contribute little towards the heritability of cancer. The genetic basis of cancers is far from being completely dissected.

One of the most notable successes of GWAS is that the majority of the genetic loci implicated for cancers have never been expected previously. In some cases, cancer low-risk loci seem to affect expression of the nearest gene in tumor tissue. In other studies, SNPs appear to be located on distant-acting transcriptional enhancers. In fact, the functional significance of most SNPs remains to be elucidated. They are likely to be the surrogate markers pointing to the loci harboring real disease causal variants.

References

Agúndez JA. N-acetyltransferases: lessons learned from eighty years of research. *Curr Drug Metab.* 2008 Jul;9(6):463-4.

Amin KS, Banerjee PP. The cellular functions of RASSF1A and its inactivation in prostate cancer. *J Carcinog.* 2012;11:3.

Bai Y, Edamatsu H, Maeda S, Saito H, Suzuki N, Satoh T, Kataoka T. Crucial role of phospholipase Cepsilon in chemical carcinogen-induced skin tumor development. *Cancer Res.* 2004 Dec 15;64(24):8808-10.

Baird DM. Variation at the TERT locus and predisposition for cancer. *Expert Rev Mol Med.* 2010 May 18;12:e16.

Bellam N, Pasche B. Tgf-beta signaling alterations and colon cancer. *Cancer Treat Res.* 2010;155:85-103.

Birts CN, Bergman LM, Blaydes JP. CtBPs promote mitotic fidelity through their activities in the cell nucleus. *Oncogene.* 2011 Mar 17;30(11):1272-80.

Broeks A, Schmidt MK, Sherman ME, Couch FJ, Hopper JL, Dite GS, Apicella C, Smith LD, Hammet F, Southey MC, et al. Low penetrance breast cancer susceptibility loci are associated with specific breast tumor subtypes: findings from the Breast Cancer Association Consortium. *Hum Mol Genet.* 2011 Aug 15;20(16):3289-303.

Campa D, Kaaks R, Le Marchand L, Haiman CA, Travis RC, Berg CD, Buring JE, Chanock SJ, Diver WR, Dostal L, et al. Interactions between genetic variants and breast cancer risk factors in the breast and prostate cancer cohort consortium. *J Natl Cancer Inst.* 2011 Aug 17;103(16):1252-63.

Chen L, Hong C, Chen EC, Yee SW, Xu L, Almof EU, Wen C, Fujii K, Johns SJ, Stryke D, et al. Genetic and epigenetic regulation of the organic cation transporter 3, SLC22A3. *Pharmacogenomics J.* 2012 Jan 10.

Choi W, Shah JB, Tran M, Svatek R, Marquis L, Lee IL, Yu D, Adam L, Wen S, Shen Y, et al. p63 expression defines a lethal subset of muscle-invasive bladder cancers. *PLoS One.* 2012;7(1):e30206.

Ciampa J, Yeager M, Amundadottir L, Jacobs K, Kraft P, Chung C, Wacholder S, Yu K, Wheeler W, Thun MJ, et al. Large-scale exploration of gene-gene interactions in prostate cancer using a multistage genome-wide association study. *Cancer Res.* 2011 May 1;71(9):3287-95.

Easton DF, Pooley KA, Dunning AM, Pharoah PD, Thompson D, Ballinger DG, Struewing JP, Morrison J, Field H, Luben R, et al. Genome-wide association study identifies novel breast cancer susceptibility loci. *Nature.* 2007 Jun 28;447(7148):1087-93.

Fanale D, Amodeo V, Corsini LR, Rizzo S, Bazan V, Russo A. Breast cancer genome-wide association studies: there is strength in numbers. *Oncogene.* 2012 Apr 26;31(17):2121-8.

Garcia-Closas M, Hall P, Nevanlinna H, Pooley K, Morrison J, Richesson DA, Bojesen SE, Nordestgaard BG, Axelsson CK, Arias JI, et al. Heterogeneity of breast cancer associations with five susceptibility loci by clinical and pathological characteristics. *PLoS Genet.* 2008 Apr 25;4(4):e1000054.

Goode EL, Chenevix-Trench G, Song H, Ramus SJ, Notaridou M, Lawrenson K, Widschwendter M, Vierkant RA, Larson MC, Kjaer SK, et al. A genome-wide association study identifies susceptibility loci for ovarian cancer at 2q31 and 8q24. *Nat Genet.* 2010 Oct;42(10):874-9.

Gutschner T, Diederichs S. The Hallmarks of Cancer: A long non-coding RNA point of view. *RNA Biol.* 2012 Jun 1;9(6).

Habbig S, Bartram MP, Müller RU, Schwarz R, Andriopoulos N, Chen S, Sägmüller JG, Hoehne M, Burst V, Liebau MC, et al. NPHP4, a cilia-associated protein, negatively regulates the Hippo pathway. J Cell Biol. 2011 May 16;193(4):633-42.

Hein R, Maranian M, Hopper JL, Kapuscinski MK, Southey MC, Park DJ, Schmidt MK, Broeks A, Hogervorst FB, Bueno-de-Mesquit HB, et al. Comparison of 6q25 Breast Cancer Hits from Asian and European Genome Wide Association Studies in the Breast Cancer Association Consortium (BCAC). *PLoS One.* 2012;7(8):e42380.

Hindorff LA, Gillanders EM, Manolio TA. Genetic architecture of cancer and other complex diseases: lessons learned and future directions. *Carcinogenesis.* 2011 Jul;32(7):945-54.

Huppi K, Pitt JJ, Wahlberg BM, Caplen NJ. The 8q24 gene desert: an oasis of non-coding transcriptional activity. *Front Genet.* 2012;3:69.

Jaeger E, Leedham S, Lewis A, Segditsas S, Becker M, Cuadrado PR, Davis H, Kaur K, Heinimann K, Howarth K, et al. Hereditary mixed polyposis syndrome is caused by a 40-kb upstream duplication that leads to increased and ectopic expression of the BMP antagonist GREM1. *Nat Genet.* 2012 May 6;44(6):699-703.

James MA, Wen W, Wang Y, Byers LA, Heymach JV, Coombes KR, Girard L, Minna J, You M. Functional characterization of CLPTM1L as a lung cancer risk candidate gene in the 5p15.33 locus. *PLoS One.* 2012;7(6):e36116.

Kamat AM, Mathew P. Bladder cancer: imperatives for personalized medicine. *Oncology (Williston Park).* 2011 Sep;25(10):951-8, 960.

Kashuba VI, Pavlova TV, Grigorieva EV, Kutsenko A, Yenamandra SP, Li J, Wang F, Protopopov AI, Zabarovska VI, Senchenko V, et al. High mutability of the tumor suppressor genes RASSF1 and RBSP3 (CTDSPL) in cancer. *PLoS One.* 2009 May 29;4(5):e5231.

Koboldt DC, Zhang Q, Larson DE, Shen D, McLellan MD, Lin L, Miller CA, Mardis ER, Ding L, Wilson RK. VarScan 2: somatic mutation and copy number alteration discovery in cancer by exome sequencing. *Genome Res.* 2012 Mar;22(3):568-76.

Kote-Jarai Z, Amin Al Olama A, Leongamornlert D, Tymrakiewicz M, Saunders E, Guy M, Giles GG, Severi G, Southey M, Hopper JL, et al. Identification of a novel prostate cancer susceptibility variant in the KLK3 gene transcript. *Hum Genet.* 2011 Jun;129(6):687-94.

Krimpenfort P, Ijpenberg A, Song JY, van der Valk M, Nawijn M, Zevenhoven J, Berns A. p15Ink4b is a critical tumour suppressor in the absence of p16Ink4a. *Nature.* 2007 Aug 23;448(7156):943-6.

Li Y, Sheu CC, Ye Y, de Andrade M, Wang L, Chang SC, Aubry MC, Aakre JA, Allen MS, Chen F, et al. Genetic variants and risk of lung cancer in never smokers: a genome-wide association study. *Lancet Oncol.* 2010 Apr;11(4):321-30.

Lindström S, Vachon CM, Li J, Varghese J, Thompson D, Warren R, Brown J, Leyland J, Audley T, Wareham NJ, et al. Common variants in ZNF365 are associated with both mammographic density and breast cancer risk. *Nat Genet.* 2011 Mar;43(3):185-7.

Liu Y, Liu P, Wen W, James MA, Wang Y, Bailey-Wilson JE, Amos CI, Pinney SM, Yang P, de Andrade M, et al. Haplotype and cell proliferation analyses of candidate lung cancer susceptibility genes on chromosome 15q24-25.1. *Cancer Res.* 2009 Oct 1;69(19):7844-50.

Liu Z, Wu J, Yu X. CCDC98 targets BRCA1 to DNA damage sites. *Nat Struct Mol Biol.* 2007 Aug;14(8):716-20.

Lynam-Lennon N, Reynolds JV, Marignol L, Sheils OM, Pidgeon GP, Maher SG. MicroRNA-31 modulates tumour sensitivity to radiation in oesophageal adenocarcinoma. *J Mol Med (Berl).* 2012 Jun 17.

Marafioti T, Jabri L, Pulford K, Brousset P, Mason DY, Delsol G. Leucocyte-specific protein (LSP1) in malignant lymphoma and Hodgkin's disease. *Br J Haematol.* 2003 Feb;120(4):671-8.

Melino G. p63 is a suppressor of tumorigenesis and metastasis interacting with mutant p53. *Cell Death Differ.* 2011 Sep;18(9):1487-99.

Mocellin S, Verdi D, Pooley KA, Landi MT, Egan KM, Baird DM, Prescott J, De Vivo I, Nitti D. Telomerase reverse transcriptase locus polymorphisms and cancer risk: a field synopsis and meta-analysis. *J Natl Cancer Inst.* 2012 Jun 6;104(11):840-54.

Okita K, Motohashi S, Shinnakasu R, Nagato K, Yamasaki K, Sato Y, Kitamura H, Hijikata A, Yamashita M, Shimizu K, et al. A set of genes associated with the interferon-γ response of lung cancer patients undergoing α-galactosylceramide-pulsed dendritic cell therapy. *Cancer Sci.* 2010 Nov;101(11):2333-40.

Rafnar T, Sulem P, Stacey SN, Geller F, Gudmundsson J, Sigurdsson A, Jakobsdottir M, Helgadottir H, Thorlacius S, Aben KK, et al. Sequence variants at the TERT-CLPTM1L locus associate with many cancer types. *Nat Genet.* 2009 Feb;41(2):221-7.

Riaz M, Berns EM, Sieuwerts AM, Ruigrok-Ritstier K, de Weerd V, Groenewoud A, Uitterlinden AG, Look MP, Klijn JG, Sleijfer S, et al. Correlation of breast cancer susceptibility loci with patient characteristics, metastasis-free survival, and mRNA expression of the nearest genes. *Breast Cancer Res Treat.* 2012 Jun;133(3):843-51.

Saeki N, Gu J, Yoshida T, Wu X. Prostate stem cell antigen: a Jekyll and Hyde molecule? *Clin Cancer Res.* 2010 Jul 15;16(14):3533-8.

Slattery ML, Lundgreen A, Herrick JS, Kadlubar S, Caan BJ, Potter JD, Wolff RK. Genetic variation in bone morphogenetic protein and colon and rectal cancer. *Int J Cancer.* 2012 Feb 1;130(3):653-64.

Smid M, Wang Y, Klijn JG, Sieuwerts AM, Zhang Y, Atkins D, Martens JW, Foekens JA. Genes associated with breast cancer metastatic to bone. *J Clin Oncol.* 2006 May 20;24(15):2261-7.

Stevens KN, Vachon CM, Lee AM, Slager S, Lesnick T, Olswold C, Fasching PA, Miron P, Eccles D, Carpenter JE, et al. Common breast cancer susceptibility loci are associated with triple-negative breast cancer. *Cancer Res.* 2011 Oct 1;71(19):6240-9.

Strassburg CP, Kalthoff S, Ehmer U. Variability and function of family 1 uridine-5'-diphosphate glucuronosyltransferases (UGT1A). *Crit Rev Clin Lab Sci.* 2008;45(6):485-530.

Takatsuno Y, Mimori K, Yamamoto K, Sato T, Niida A, Inoue H, Imoto S, Kawano S, Yamaguchi R, Toh H, et al. The rs6983267 SNP Is Associated with MYC Transcription Efficiency, Which Promotes Progression and Worsens Prognosis of Colorectal Cancer. *Ann Surg Oncol.* 2012 Sep 14.

Tamimi RM, Cox D, Kraft P, Colditz GA, Hankinson SE, Hunter DJ. Breast cancer susceptibility loci and mammographic density. *Breast Cancer Res.* 2008;10(4):R66.

Tarleton HP, Lemischka IR. Delayed differentiation in embryonic stem cells and mesodermal progenitors in the absence of CtBP2. *Mech Dev.* 2010 Jan-Feb;127(1-2):107-19.

Vachon CM, Scott CG, Fasching PA, Hall P, Tamimi RM, Li J, Stone J, Apicella C, Odefrey F, Gierach GL, et al. Common Breast Cancer Susceptibility Variants in LSP1 and RAD51L1 Are Associated with Mammographic Density Measures that Predict Breast Cancer Risk. *Cancer Epidemiol Biomarkers Prev.* 2012 Jul;21(7):1156-66.

Varghese JS, Easton DF. Genome-wide association studies in common cancers--what have we learnt? *Curr Opin Genet Dev.* 2010 Jun;20(3):201-9.

Wang X, Zbou C, Qiu G, Fan J, Tang H, Peng Z. Screening of new tumor suppressor genes in sporadic colorectal cancer patients. *Hepatogastroenterology.* 2008 Nov-Dec;55(88):2039-44.

Whitaker HC, Kote-Jarai Z, Ross-Adams H, Warren AY, Burge J, George A, Bancroft E, Jhavar S, Leongamornlert D, Tymrakiewicz M, et al. The rs10993994 risk allele for prostate cancer results in clinically relevant changes in microseminoprotein-beta expression in tissue and urine. *PLoS One.* 2010 Oct 13;5(10):e13363

Yamamoto K, Okamoto A, Isonishi S, Ochiai K, Ohtake Y. A novel gene, CRR9, which was up-regulated in CDDP-resistant ovarian tumor cell line, was associated with apoptosis. *Biochem Biophys Res Commun.* 2001 Feb 2;280(4):1148-54.

Yang Y, Wang F, Shi C, Zou Y, Qin H, Ma Y. Cyclin D1 G870A polymorphism contributes to colorectal cancer susceptibility: evidence from a systematic review of 22 case-control studies. *PLoS One.* 2012;7(5):e36813.

Zhang PJ, Hu XY, Liu CY, Chen ZB, Ni NN, Yu Y, Yang LN, Huang ZQ, Liu QW, Jiang AL. The inhibitory effects of NKX3.1 on IGF-1R expression and its signalling pathway in human prostatic carcinoma PC3 cells. *Asian J Androl.* 2012 May;14(3):493-8.

Zhang WB, Zhang JH, Pan ZQ, Yang QS, Liu B. The MTHFR C677T Polymorphism and Prostate Cancer Risk: New Findings from a Meta-analysis of 7306 Cases and 8062 Controls. *Asian Pac J Cancer Prev.* 2012;13(6):2597-604.

Chapter 5

Familial Cancer Syndromes

Abstract

While most cancers are sporadic, there are familial syndromes associated to the inheritance of an altered gene. This leads to a higher risk of developing a specific set of characteristic cancers, depending on the syndrome and its specifically-associated altered gene. Examples of familial cancer syndromes include ataxia telangiectasia, hereditary breast/ovarian cancer, Li-Fraumeni syndrome, Peutz-Jeghers syndrome and von Hippel-Lindau syndrome.

Introduction

Approximately 5–10% of all cancers are inherited, the majority in an autosomal dominant manner. Cancer may be associated with a wide range of hereditary disorders. Over 100 of these hereditary cancer susceptibility syndromes have been described.

The presence of a hereditary cancer predisposition is suggested by various features in the individual patient and in the patient's family (Weber et al. 2001).

In the individual patient, these features may be:

- Multiple primary tumors in the same organ
- Multiple primary tumors in different organs
- Bilateral primary tumors in paired organs
- Multifocality within a single organ
- Younger-than-usual age at tumor diagnosis
- Rare histology
- In the sex not usually affected
- Associated with other genetic traits
- Associated with congenital defects
- Associated with an inherited precursor lesion
- Associated with another rare disease
- Associated with cutaneous lesions known to be related to
- cancer susceptibility disorders (eg, the genodermatoses)

In the patient's family, features are:

- One first-degree relative with the same or a related tumor and
- one of the individual features listed
- ≥ two first-degree relatives with tumors of the same site
- ≥ two first-degree relatives with tumor types belonging to a
- known familial cancer syndrome
- ≥ two first-degree relatives with rare tumors
- ≥ two relatives in two generations with tumors of the same site
- or etiologically related sites

Some familial cancer syndromes show autosomal dominant inheritance. In such a case, an affected person has a 50% chance of passing on the genetic mutation to each of his or her children. Other familial cancer syndromes show autosomal recessive inheritance, which means that both parents are usually not affected, but are carriers of a mutation for the condition. In autosomal recessive inheritance, each child born to parents who are carriers has a 25% chance of having the condition.

A List of Cancer-Prone Diseases

Ataxia Telangiectasia (ATM) (Includes Complementation Groups A, C, D, E)

- **ATM** (Basu et al. 2012) is a primary immunodeficiency disease that affects a number of different organs in the body. It is characterized by neurological problems, particularly abnormalities of balance, recurrent sinus and respiratory infections, and dilated blood vessels in the eyes and on the surface of the skin. Patients usually have immune system abnormalities and are very sensitive to the effects of radiation treatments.
- **Incidence**: one ATM case in 30,000 to one in 100,000 live births; heterozygosity in the general population is estimated to about 0.2%–1.0%.
- **Inheritance pattern**: autosomal recessive.
- **Gene and chromosomal location**: ATM at 11q22.3. It encodes a large serine-threonine kinase mediating cell cycle arrest in response to ionizing radiation through the phosphorylation of targets including p53, BRCA1 and CHEK2.
- Complementation groups are defined on the basis of a characteristic radioresistant DNA replication phenotype as a marker in cultured cells. Four complementation groups—A, C, D, and E—map to the same locus and show the following distribution worldwide: A = 55%, C = 28%, D = 14% and E = 3%.
- **Mutations**: a variety of germinal ATM mutations have been reported, with 70%–85% resulting in a truncated protein. These mutations are dispersed throughout the gene, and therefore most patients are compound heterozygotes; however, most mutations appear to inactivate the ATM protein by truncation, large deletions, or

annulation of initiation or termination. Missense mutations have been described in breast cancer patients, but do not seem to contribute to ataxia telangiectasia.
- **Associated malignant neoplasms**: one-third of all ATM patients will develop cancer, and 15% will die of cancer. Milder, clinically atypical forms of ATM have been identified. Eighty-five percent of the associated malignant neoplasms involve lymphoreticular tissue, especially non-Hodgkin lymphoma (usually B-cell), a feature shared by other disorders exhibiting immunodeficiency, and leukemia (usually acute or chronic lymphocytic leukemia). Adult male patients, particularly those who are IgA deficient, have a 70-fold increased risk of gastric cancer. Increased rates of medulloblastomas, basal cell carcinomas, gliomas, and uterine cancers have been reported. Most people with ATM live into their 30s with cancer and infection accounting for 90% of mortality.
- **Associated benign neoplasms**: none known.

Basal Cell Nevus Syndrome (BCNS)

- **BCNS** (Lo Muzio 2008) is a disease characterized by multiple basal cell skin cancers or basal cell nevus syndrome. Other common findings include jaw cysts, pits on the palms of the hands or soles of the feet, calcium deposits in soft tissues, and skeletal (bone) changes.
- **Incidence**: estimated at one in 40,000–57,000 live births.
- **Inheritance pattern**: autosomal dominant.
- **Gene and chromosomal location**: PTCH1 at 9q22.3. It encodes a member of the patched gene family and is the receptor for sonic hedgehog, a secreted molecule implicated in the formation of embryonic structures and in tumorigenesis.
- **Mutations**: multiple unique PTCH1 mutations have been reported, but no clinically significant genotype–phenotype correlations were noted. Mutations are detected in 60%–85% of individuals meeting diagnostic criteria. Twenty to forty percent of cases represent de novo germline mutations. Rarely, cytogenetically detectable deletions of chromosome 9q have been reported.
- **Associated malignant neoplasms**: multiple basal cell carcinomas (BCC) usually appear in the third decade, but have been reported as young as age 2 years, with a median age at diagnosis of 25 years. Ten percent of gene mutation carriers may never develop BCC. Up to 5% of children develop medulloblastoma with a peak incidence around age 2 years, compared with 7 years in sporadic medulloblastomas. Ovarian fibrosarcoma has been observed.
- **Associated benign neoplasms**: odontogenic keratocysts of the jaw in over 90% of individuals with BCNS, often developing in the second decade, and epidermal cysts and palmoplantar pits reportedly occur in the majority of cases. In a minority of cases, meningioma or ovarian fibromas and cardiac fibromas may occur. Fetal rhabdomyomas have been reported now in five cases.

Beckwith–Wiedemann Syndrome (BWS) (Exomphalos–Macroglossia–Gigantism Syndrome)

- **BWS** (Choufani et al. 2010) is a growth disorder characterized by macrosomia, macroglossia, visceromegaly, embryonal tumors, omphalocele, neonatal hypoglycemia, ear creases/pits, adrenocortical cytomegaly, and renal abnormalities.
- **Incidence**: one BWS case in 13,700 live births. Children conceived through *in vitro* fertilization (IVF) have a three to fourfold increased chance of developing BWS. This is probably due to genes being turned on or off by the IVF procedures
- **Inheritance pattern**: autosomal dominant pattern is seen in less than 15% of cases. Inheritance is mostly maternal (imprinting) with a more severe phenotype after maternal transmission. More than 85% of cases have no family history of BWS.
- **Genes and chromosomal location**: some BWS patients have maternal chromosomal rearrangements of 11p15, meaning that there is a disruption of the chromosome in this region. Other patients have paternal uniparental disomy of chromosome 11, meaning that the maternal copy of this chromosome is replaced with an extra paternal copy. Many other patients have abnormal DNA methylation in different areas of 11p15, meaning that normal epigenetic marks that regulate imprinted (they are expressed differently depending on whether they came from the mother or father - only one parental copy is active) genes in this region are altered. At least five different genes in the 11p15 region have been implicated in the etiology of BWS: IGF2, H19, KVLQT1, LIT1 and KCNQ1OT1. Additionally, even after extensive molecular testing, the specific defect causing BWS in an affected individual may remain unknown. In about 1/3 of BWS patients, the genetic or epigenetic mutation is unknown. This fact demonstrates why BWS remains a clinical diagnosis because physicians cannot identify and test for all the genetic causes of BWS.
- **Associated malignant neoplasms**: while most children with BWS do not develop cancer, they have a 7.5% risk of tumors (all sites combined) in the first 8 years of life; development of cancer above that age is uncommon. The most common neoplasm is Wilms tumor. The contralateral kidney is also affected in 21% of BWS-related Wilms tumor. Other BWS-associated tumors include adrenocortical carcinoma, rhabdomyosarcoma, hepatoblastoma, neuroblastoma, and gonadoblastoma.
- **Associated benign neoplasms**: pancreatic islet cell hyperplasia (leading to neonatal hypoglycemia), adrenal cytomegaly (which may or may not result in adrenal overactivity), hyperplasia of pituitary, hamartomas, adenomas, myxomas, ganglioneuromas, and fibroadenomas.

Birt–Hogg–Dubé Syndrome (BHDS)

- **BHDS** (Maher 2011) involves cutaneous manifestations (fibrofolliculomas, trichodiscomas, angiofibromas, perifollicular fibromas, and acrochordons), pulmonary cysts/history of pneumothorax, and various types of renal tumors.

- **Incidence**: unknown. BHDS is considered to be rare, and sometimes estimated to 1 in 200,000 people.
- **Inheritance pattern**: autosomal dominant.
- **Gene and chromosomal location**: FLCN (folliculin) at 17p11.2. Although its precise in vivo function is unknown, folliculin appears involved in AMPK and mTOR signaling.
- **Mutations**: about 50% of BHDS-related FLCN mutations involve an insertion or deletion of a C-8 hypermutable tract in exon 11; other mutations are found throughout the gene. Overall, FLCN sequence analysis has an 84% detection rate in BHDS.
- **Associated malignant neoplasms**: BHDS is associated with multiple bilateral renal tumors of various types, including oncocytoma, chromophobe renal cell carcinoma, clear cell carcinoma, and papillary renal carcinoma, as well as hybrid oncocytic neoplasms. Nonrenal malignancies are not known to be part of this syndrome.
- **Associated benign neoplasms**: benign tumors of the hair follicle, including follicular fibromas, perifollicular fibromas, trichodiscomas, and acrochordons. Other features of BHDS include pulmonary cysts and, rarely, deforming lipomas and collagenomas.

Bloom Syndrome (BS) (Bloom–Torre–Machacek Syndrome)

- **BS** (Monnat 2010) is characterized by severe pre- and postnatal growth deficiency, highly characteristic sparseness of subcutaneous fat tissue throughout infancy and early childhood, and short stature throughout postnatal life which in most affected individuals is accompanied by an erythematous and sun-sensitive skin lesion of the face. Gastroesophageal reflux is common and very possibly responsible for infections of the upper respiratory tract, the middle ear, and the lung that occur repeatedly in most persons with BS.
- **Incidence**: actual incidence is unknown in general population. Only a few hundred cases have been reported so far. However, among Ashkenazi Jews, Bloom syndrome (BS) is seen in one in 48,000 live births and is most common in those of Ukrainian or Polish ancestry.
- **Inheritance pattern**: autosomal recessive. High penetrance.
- **Gene and chromosomal location**: BLM at 15q26.1. Like WRN in Werner Syndrome, BLM is a RecQlike DNA helicase maybe contributing to telomere maintenance.
- **Mutations**: multiple mutations have been identified, including missense, nonsense, frameshift, exon skipping, and exonic deletions. Nineteen different recurring (founder) mutations were reported.
- **Associated malignant neoplasms**: cancers show increased frequency at all ages, with acute leukemia, lymphoid neoplasms, and Wilms tumor predominating before the age of 25; after age 20, carcinomas of the tongue, larynx, lung, esophagus, colon, skin, breast, and cervix are most frequent.

- **Associated benign neoplasms**: multiple adenomatous colon polyps have been reported in one individual with BS.

Carney Complex, Types I and II (CNC1 and CNC2)

- **CNC** (Shetty Roy et al. 2011) is a condition comprising myxomas of the heart and skin, hyperpigmentation of the skin (lentiginosis), and endocrine overactivity.
- **Incidence**: rare. Exact incidence is unknown.
- **Inheritance pattern**: autosomal dominant.
- **Gene and chromosomal location**: Carney complex type 1 (CNC1) is due to mutations in PRKAR1A at 17q22–q24, detected in about 50%–65% of CNC cases and in a subset of patients with isolated primary pigmented nodular adrenocortical dysplasia (PPNAD) (see below). PRKAR1A is a tumor suppressor gene that codes for the protein kinase A regulatory 1-alpha subunit. A subset of families (approximately 30%) with CNC have been linked to chromosomal band 2p16 (CNC2), but the gene has not been identified.
- **Mutations**: the majority of PRKAR1A mutations are nonsense, frameshift and splicesite mutations, leading to a truncated protein. Large deletions were also recently reported. Mutations are primarily seen in two hotspots, delTG576-577 and C769T.
- **Associated malignant neoplasms**: testicular tumors occur in one-third of boys with CNC and nearly all adult males. The tumors are large cell calcifying Sertoli cell tumors (LCCSTs) and Leydig cell tumors. A syndrome-related predisposition to pancreatic cancer is likely.
- **Associated benign neoplasms**: the skin is the most commonly affected organ, with about 80% of patients presenting one or more skin lesions: lentigines, compound nevi, blue nevi, café-au-lait macules, or cutaneous myxoma. Spotty cutaneous pigmentation is common, especially involving the face, eyelids, vermillion border of lips, conjunctiva, sclera, vulva, glans penis, back of hands, and feet. Cardiac myxomas are observed in a majority of patients and are multiple in half of cases. Myxoid uterine leiomyomas also occur. PPNAD, with or without overt Cushing syndrome, is the most common endocrine manifestation of CNC, reported in 30%–40% of cases. Pituitary adenomas are found in about 10% of patients. Thyroid adenomas are occasionally observed. The presence of a calcifying pigmented neuroectodermal tumor (psammomatous melanotic schwannoma) is highly characteristic of CNC; it occurs in about 10% of patients. Breast duct adenomas, breast myxomas, and osteochondromyxomas of bone also occur.

Cowden Syndrome

- **CS** (Zbuk and Eng 2007) is a disease characterized by a high risk of both benign and cancerous tumors of the breast, thyroid, and endometrium. Other key features of CS

are skin changes (such as trichilemmomas and papillomatous papules) and macrocephaly.
- **Incidence**: estimated to one in 200,000 to one in 250,000 live births.
- **Inheritance pattern**: autosomal dominant.
- **Gene and chromosomal location**: PTEN at 10q23.3. A tumor suppressor gene, PTEN encodes a phosphatase with tumor suppressive effects, negative regulator of the PI3K/Akt signal cell pathway by dephosphorylating PIP3. G_1 cell cycle arrest and/or apoptosis result, depending on the tissue type.
- **Mutations**: mutations in PTEN have been found in 80% of CS patients. Haplotype analysis suggests that mutation-negative patients may harbor deleterious PTEN mutations that are not detected by standard genetic testing methods. In PTEN sequencing-negative, clinically positive CS, approximately 10% have large deletions and approximately 10% have promoter mutations, which require alternate analytic techniques for their detection.
- **Associated malignant neoplasms**: female breast cancer (up to 30% of CS women), occurring about 10 years younger than in the general population Male breast cancer also can occur. There is an elevated lifetime risk of thyroid cancer (mainly follicular less frequently papillary) (reported in 15% of the patients) and an increased risk of endometrial and renal cancers.
- **Associated benign neoplasms**: verrucous skin lesions of the face (trichilemmomas) and limbs (hyperkeratoses) and oral papillomatosis with cobblestone gingival. Hamartomatous polyps of the stomach, small bowel, and colon. Lipomas, cerebellar gangliocytomatosis, hemangiomas, and multiple early-onset uterine leiomyomas are common in CS.

Dyskeratosis Congenita (DC) (Zinsser Cole Engeman Syndrome, Hoyeraal Hreidarsson Syndrome)

- DC (Mason and Bessler 2011) is a syndrome associated with abnormal shapes to fingernails and toenails, a lacy rash on the face and chest, and white patches in the mouth. More than half of the patients are males. About half of DC patients develop bone marrow failure.
- **Incidence**: rare
- **Inheritance pattern**: predominantly X-linked recessive (>50%); autosomal dominant (5%), recessive (10%), or undetermined inheritance also occur.
- **Gene and chromosomal location**: X-linked recessive dyskeratosis congenita (DC) is due to mutations in DKC1, Xq28, which encodes the protein, dyskerin, a small nucleolar RNA functionally associated with the RNA component of TERC. Autosomal dominant DC is due to telomerase RNA component, hTR/TERC, 3q21–q28 or to telomerase reverse transcriptase, TERT, 5p15.33. Biallelic mutations in TERT have been associated with an autosomal recessive or apparently sporadic pattern of DC. NOP10 (NOLA3), 15q14–q15, has been implicated as the etiologic basis of DC in one large consanguineous family (3). It produces a protein component

of H/ACA snoRNP complexes that include telomerase and dyskerin. TINF2, 14q11.2, a component of the telomere-related shelterin complex, has been recently identified as a new, autosomal dominant, DC gene. All these genes identified as predisposing to DC are members of the telomere maintenance pathway and together account for approximately 75% of all DC families.
- **Mutations**: in families with X-linked DC, the majority of mutations in DKC1 result in single amino acid substitutions in the dyskerin protein. One mutation, causing an alanine-to-valine substitution at position 353, accounts for 30% of X-linked DC, and it can arise as a de novo event. No genotype–phenotype correlations have been observed with specific mutations. Mutations in TERC include large intragenic and terminal deletions, a small frameshift mutation, and point mutations often resulting in haploinsufficiency for functional telomerase. These mutations do not account for all autosomal dominant DC. TERC deletions are associated with progressive telomere shortening, resulting in clinical anticipation with more severe disease presenting at an earlier age in successive generations.
- **Associated malignant neoplasms**: they are reported in approximately 10% of patients. They include acute myelogenous leukemia (AML) and carcinomas of the upper aerodigestive tract, particularly squamous cell cancers of the head and neck and esophagus.
- **Associated benign neoplasms**: myelodysplasia, in patients with bone marrow failure, may precede the development of AML. Leukoplakia commonly affects the oral mucosa and may evolve into squamous cell carcinoma. Leukoplakia occasionally is found in conjunctiva, urethra, or genital mucosa. Predisposition to fibrosis in DC may present as symptomatic esophageal or urethral stenosis.

Familial Adenomatous Polyposis (FAP)

- **FAP** (Half et al. 2009) is characterized by the development of hundreds to thousands of adenomatous polyps throughout the colon and rectum, with an extremely high lifetime risk of colon cancer. The clinical diagnosis of FAP is made if an individual has greater than 100 colorectal adenomas
- **Incidence**: about 1 in every 5000–10 000 people. The frequency of gene mutations in the general population is unknown.
- **Inheritance pattern**: autosomal dominant. Penetrance is almost complete.
- **Gene and chromosomal location**: APC at 5q21–q22. APC binds to β-catenin and targets it for degradation by the cell. This, in turn, prevents β-catenin from entering the nucleus and participating in the Tcf-mediated transcription of a number of target genes, including MYC. APC is also critical for the stabilization of microtubule–kinetochore interactions. Thus, inactivation of APC may contribute to chromosomal instability (CIN) and an enhanced mutation rate, promoting tumor growth in colorectal cancer.
- **Mutations**: protein truncation mutations comprise 70%–80% of mutations, and approximately 25% of cases represent new germline mutations. Attenuated polyposis (<100 polyps) is correlated with mutations before codon 157, after codon 1595, and in the alternatively spliced region of exon 9. Mutations between codons 1250 and

1464 correlate with severe polyposis (>1000 polyps). Mutations in other areas have an intermediate polyp phenotype. Desmoid tumors are associated with mutations after codon 1444. No consistent correlations were found for upper gastrointestinal tumors.
- **Associated malignant neoplasms**: they include colon adenocarcinoma; duodenal carcinomas, especially around the ampulla of Vater; follicular or papillary thyroid cancer occurs in about 2% of affected individuals. The risk of childhood hepatoblastoma is estimated 0.6%; it is rare after age 6 years. Germline mutations in APC were found in 10% of 50 cases of apparently sporadic hepatoblastomas. The lifetime risk of pancreatic cancer is 2%, and this may include islet cell tumors. Some FAP families have brain tumors, of which 60% are medulloblastomas (gliomas and ependymomas also reported).
- **Associated benign neoplasms**: FAP includes numerous non-malignant neoplasms: adenomatous polyps of the colon, duodenal polyps (especially periampullary), hamartomatous gastric polyps, adenomatous gastric polyps. Dental abnormalities including supernumerary or congenitally absent teeth, dentigerous cysts, and osteomas of the jaw are also seen in individuals with FAP. Other benign lesions include sebaceous or epidermoid cysts, lipomas, and congenital hypertrophy of the retinal pigment epithelium. Osteomas may arise in any bone. Desmoid tumors—histologically benign clonal neoplasms comprised of fibrous tissue—cause substantial morbidity and mortality in approximately 5% of FAP patients.

Familial Platelet Disorder with Predisposition to Acute Myelogenous Leukemia (FPD/AML)

- **FPD/AML** (Segel and Lichtman 2004) is a disorder characterized by qualitative and quantitative platelet defects, and propensity to develop acute myelogenous leukemia (AML).
- **Incidence**: very rare.
- **Inheritance pattern**: autosomal dominant. Complete penetrance.
- **Gene and chromosomal location**: RUNX1 (previously CBFA2), at 21q22.3. It encodes a transcription factor that regulates the differentiation of hematopoietic stem cells into mature blood cells.
- **Mutations**: RUNX1 mutations appear to result in haploinsufficiency.
- **Associated malignant neoplasms**: population studies suggest an increased risk of hematologic malignancies in families of children with acute myeloid leukemias and a trend toward increased risks of solid tumors that did not reach statistical significance.
- **Associated benign neoplasms**: none described.

Fanconi Anemia (FA)

- **FA** (Su and Huang 2011) is a disease characterized by chromosomal instability, bone marrow failure, cancer susceptibility, and a profound sensitivity to agents that produce DNA interstrand cross-link.

- **Incidence**: estimated to 1 case per 350,000 births
- **Inheritance pattern**: autosomal recessive except FANCB, which is X-linked recessive. High penetrance.
- **Genes and chromosomal locations**: There are at least 14 genes whose mutations are known to cause FA: see table 1

Table 1. Fanconi anemia genetics

Gene	Chromosome	FA complementation group
FANCA	16q24.3	A
FANCB/FAAP95	Xp22.31	B
FANCC	9q22.3	C
FANCD1/BRCA2	13q12.3	D1
FANCD2	3p25.3	D2
FANCE	6p21–p22	E
FANCF	11p15	F
FANCG/XRCC9	9p13	G
FANCI/KIAA1794	15q25–q26	I
FANCJ/BACH1/BRIP1	17q22–q24	J
FANCL/PHF9/FAAP43/POG	2p16.1	L
FANCM/FAAP250/Hef	14q21.3	M
FANCN/PALB2	16p12.1	N
FANCO/RAD51C	17q25.1	O

- **Mutations**: FANCA mutations account for approximately 66% of all cases; FANCC and FANCG together account for approximately 9% each; FANCD1, FANCD2, FANCE, and FANCF each account for approximately 2%–3%; and the remaining groups (FANCB, FANCI, FANCJ, FANCL, FANCM, FANCN = PALB), less than 1% each.
- **Associated malignant neoplasms**: acute myeloid leukemia; hepatocellular carcinoma; squamous cell cancer of the head, neck, and esophagus; vulvar and cervical cancer in women; and brain tumors.
- **Associated benign neoplasms**: hepatic adenomas.

Hereditary Breast/Ovarian Cancer (HBOC)

- **HBOC** (Marshall and Solomon 2007) is a syndrome that predispose to breast and ovarian cancers.
- **Incidence**: the incidence of BRCA1 mutation is between 1 in 500 and 1 in 800 in the general population; the incidence of BRCA2 mutation is even lower. However, specific groups may be characterized by a much higher risk. For instance, 1 in 40 individuals with Ashkenazi Jewish background have an increased incidence of BRCA1 and BRCA2 mutations.
- **Inheritance pattern**: autosomal dominant. BRCA1 mutation carriers had a cumulative risk of developing breast or ovarian cancer by age 70 of 65 and 39%,

respectively. For BRCA2 mutation carriers, the risks were 45% for breast cancer and 11% for ovarian cancer.
- **Genes and chromosomal location**: BRCA1, at 17q21, and BRCA2, at 13q12.3. Both encode proteins involved in repair of DNA damages.
- **Mutations**: more than 1500 distinct mutations, polymorphisms, and variants have been identified in BRCA1 and more than 1900 in BRCA2 (Breast Cancer Information Core: http://research.nhgri.nih.gov/bic/).
- **Associated malignant neoplasms**: breast and ovarian cancer are the defining features of the syndrome. The risk of BRCA-related breast and ovarian cancer appears to be confined to epithelial malignancies of both organs. BRCA1-related breast cancer tends to be of high histological grade, lymph node positive, estrogen receptor negative, progesterone receptor negative, HER2/neu negative, with expression of basal or myoepithelial markers by immunohistochemistry ("basal phenotype") (Lacroix and Leclercq 2005). Recent data indicate that the dearth of estrogen receptors in BRCA1-related breast cancer is a direct result of the mutation itself; BRCA1 regulates the expression of estrogen receptors. Whereas the clinical features of BRCA2-related breast cancer are indistinguishable from those of sporadic breast cancer, these two entities do appear to have distinctive molecular characteristics by mRNA expression profiles. The primary difference between BRCA-related ovarian cancer and sporadic ovarian cancer is the rarity of mucinous and borderline neoplasms in the former. Fallopian tube carcinoma is now a well-established component of the BRCA-related cancer spectrum. Carriers of BRCA1 mutations are at risk of primary papillary serous carcinoma of the peritoneum, a malignancy that is indistinguishable from serous epithelial ovarian carcinoma. Prostate cancer also occurs in male carriers of BRCA1 mutations. It has been suggested that this risk of prostate cancer may vary substantially, depending on the location of the BRCA1 mutation. A variety of other cancers have been inconsistently implicated as part of the BRCA1 cancer susceptibility syndromes. The most convincing associations are increased risks of pancreatic cancer and male breast cancer.
- **Associated benign neoplasms**: none known.

Notes

1. BRCA1 and BRCA2 are not the only genetic abnormalities that increase risk of breast cancer. Mutations in several other genes, including TP53, PTEN, STK11/LKB1, CDH1, CHEK2, ATM, MLH1, and MSH2, have been associated with hereditary breast and or ovarian tumors. These mutations account for only a minor fraction of hereditary breast cancers. The great majority of hereditary breast cancer occurs in carriers of BRCA1 and BRCA2. Overall, it has been estimated that inherited BRCA1 and BRCA2 mutations account for 5 to 10 percent of the total breast cancers and 10 to 15 percent of the total ovarian cancers among white women in the United States.

2. Biallelic mutations in BRCA2 have been shown to cause the D1 subtype of Fanconi Anemia. Affected individuals have extreme sensitivity to chemotherapy and therapeutic irradiation; full-dose treatment can be lethal. FANC-D1 patients have very high rates of

spontaneous chromosomal instability and are at risk of Wilms tumor and medulloblastoma as well as the more typical acute leukemia.

Hereditary Diffuse Gastric Cancer (HDGC)

- **HDGC** (Schrader and Huntsman 2010) is a condition associated with an increased risk of diffuse gastric cancer.
- **Incidence**: unknown. Among apparently sporadic cases of diffuse gastric cancer or mixed gastric cancer with diffuse component, CDH1 mutations are seldom present. About one-third of families meeting criteria (below) for HDGC have identifiable germline CDH1 mutations.
- **Inheritance pattern**: autosomal dominant.
- **Gene and chromosomal location**: CDH1 on chromosomal band 16q22.1.
- **Mutations**: as of 2004, 48 families with 45 different CDH1 germline mutations had been reported. Seventy-six percent were loss-of-function mutations.
- **Associated malignant neoplasms**: diffuse gastric cancer (average age at diagnosis: 40 years). Germline CDH1 mutations have also been reported in women with invasive lobular carcinoma who present an early age at diagnosis and/or a positive family history of breast cancer, in the absence of a personal or family history of diffuse gastric cancer
- **Associated benign neoplasms**: no benign precursor lesions have been defined. There are multiple reports of multifocal microscopic intramucosal signet ring cell adenocarcinoma in specimens from prophylactic gastrectomies on individuals with CDH1 germline mutations. No information is available regarding the age at which carcinoma in situ lesions first appear, nor the natural history of these early neoplasms, although intramucosal foci of cancer cells have been reported to remain confined to the mucosa for many years.

Hereditary Leiomyomatosis and Renal Cell Cancer (HLRCC)

- **HLRCC** (Rosner et al. 2009) is a disorder characterized by cutaneous leiomyomata (multiple or single in 76% of affected individuals), uterine leiomyomata (fibroids), and/or a single renal tumor.
- **Incidence**: very rare
- **Inheritance pattern**: autosomal dominant.
- **Gene and chromosomal location**: FH, on 1q42.1. Fumarate hydratase, the protein encoded by FH, catalyzes the conversion of fumarate to 1-malate in the mitochondrial tricarboxylic acid cycle, and thus, like SDH genes in hereditary paraganglioma, FH is important in cellular energy metabolism.
- **Mutations**: mutations in FH include missense (58%), frameshift (27%), nonsense (9%), and large deletions (7%). Loss of enzymatic activity is associated with many of these mutations.

- **Associated malignant neoplasms**: aggressive renal cell carcinoma (RCC) is the primary type of cancer reported in this disorder with a median age at diagnosis of 44 years. Six cases of "uterine leiomyosarcoma" have been reported in HLRCC families, but the risk in HLRCC is unclear.
- **Associated benign neoplasms**: multiple cutaneous and uterine leiomyomas. The cutaneous lesions have not been reported to undergo malignant degeneration.

Hereditary Multiple Exostosis (HME) (Includes Type 1, Type 2, Type 3, and Multiple Osteochondromas (Enchondromatosis))

- **HME** (Jennes et al. 2009) is associated to the development of multiple benign bone tumors called exostoses. The number of exostoses and the bones on which they are located vary greatly among affected individuals.
- **Incidence**: estimated prevalence ranges from 0.9 to 2 per 100 000 live births (in white populations). Among all individuals with chondrosarcoma, about 5% have HME.
- **Inheritance pattern**: autosomal dominant with nearly complete penetrance, especially in males.
- **Gene and chromosomal location**: EXT1, EXT2, and EXT3 are located at 8q24.11–q24.13, 11p11–p12, and 19p, respectively.
- **Mutations**: more than 80 different mutations have been reported in EXT1, which accounts for 50%–76% of families with HME. Twenty-one to fifty percent of families have mutations in EXT2. A few families link to the EXT3 locus; the gene has not been cloned—and a few are not linked to any of these three loci. About 10% of affected individuals have a de novo mutation. Overall mutation detection rate is about 85%–90%.
- **Associated malignant neoplasms**: malignant transformation to chondrosarcoma or other sarcomas occurs in less than 5% of cases. Chondrosarcoma, which has a predilection for the proximal femur or axial skeleton (80%) in HME, seldom occurs before age 10 or after age 50.
- **Associated benign neoplasms**: osteochondromas and multiple exostoses, which may cause a variety of compressive problems.

Hereditary Nonpolyposis Colon Cancer (HNPCC) (Lynch Syndrome)

- **HNPCC** (Backes and Cohn 2011) is characterized by a significantly increased risk of developing colorectal cancer and an increased risk of developing other types of cancers.

- **Incidence**: HNPCC specifically due to deleterious mutations in any one of four DNA mismatch repair genes (MLH1, MSH2, MSH6, and PMS2), accounts for 2%–3% of all colorectal cancers.
- **Inheritance pattern**: autosomal dominant. High penetrance.
- **Gene and chromosomal location**: MLH1 at 3p21.3, MSH2 at 2p21–p22, PMS2 at 7p22, MSH6 at 2p16, and, maybe, PMS1 at 2q31–q33 and MSH3 at 5q11–q12. The role of MSH3 and PMS1 in hereditary disease remains unclear. The products of these genes participate in a multimeric DNA mismatch repair (MMR) complex. Syndrome-related deleterious germline mutations have clearly been documented for MLH1, MSH2, MSH6, and PMS2.
- **Mutations**: mutations in MLH1 and MSH2 account for 75-90% of cases, with MSH6 accounting for 7-13% and PMS2 for about 10%. Large deletions and/or duplications account for 5%–10% of MLH1 mutations and more than 20% of MSH2 mutations. A database of mismatch repair gene variants of all types is available (http://www.med.mun.ca/MMRvariants/default.aspx).
- **Associated malignant neoplasms**: colorectal cancers (CRC), two-thirds of which are located in the right side of the colon, with average age at diagnosis in the mid 40s. The risk of colon cancer appears to be greater in carriers of MLH1 vs. other MMR genes, but the overall risk of all cancers combined may be greatest with MSH2 mutations. The lifetime risk of CRC is about 70% by age 70 in high-risk clinic series. The lifetime risk of endometrial adenocarcinoma is 30%–60%, with an average age at diagnosis also in the 40s. Lifetime risks of gastric, biliary tract, urinary tract, and ovarian carcinoma have been estimated as 19%, 18%, 10%, and 9%, respectively. Small bowel carcinoma is also a syndrome-related malignancy, having been reported in mutation carriers of each of the four susceptibility genes.

  MSH6 appears to have later age at diagnosis of CRCs and endometrial cancer; MSH6 germline mutations have been reported to result in higher risk of endometrial cancer (lifetime risk of approximately 70%) and lower penetrance for the other Lynch syndrome–related tumors.
- **Associated benign neoplasms**: colonic adenomas, keratoacanthomas, sebaceous adenomas, Fordyce granules (intraoral ectopic sebaceous glands), and epitheliomas.

Hereditary Papillary Renal Cell Carcinoma (HPRCC)

- **HPRCC** is a disorder characterized by an increased risk of multiple kidney tumors and an increased risk of developing tumors on both kidneys.
- **Incidence**: papillary renal cell cancer (PRCC) accounts for 15%–20% of all RCCs and occurs in both sporadic and familial forms. Among all RCC combined, approximately 2% represent familial cases. A striking male predominance has been consistently noted in sporadic but not HPRCC.
- **Inheritance pattern**: autosomal dominant.
- **Gene and chromosomal location**: MET proto-oncogene at 7q31.1–34. It encodes a membrane receptor that is essential for embryonic development and wound healing.

Abnormal MET activation in cancer correlates with poor prognosis, where aberrantly active MET triggers tumor growth, angiogenesis and metastasis.
- **Mutations**: they were originally found in four of seven families with hereditary papillary renal cell carcinoma (HPRCC); more than 30 families have now been reported worldwide.
- **Associated malignant neoplasms**: papillary renal cell cancer (PRCC). MET mutation carriers have been reported to develop gastric, rectal, lung, pancreatic, and bile duct cancers, but data are insufficient at present to determine whether gene carriers are at increased risk of specific non-RCC malignancies.
- **Associated benign neoplasms**: papillary renal adenomas may precede carcinoma development.

Hereditary Paraganglioma-Pheochromocytoma (PGL/PCC) Syndrome

- **PGL/PCC** (Müller 2011) is a disease characterized by paragangliomas and by pheochromocytomas. The risk of malignant transformation is greater for extra-adrenal sympathetic paragangliomas than for pheochromocytomas or head and neck paragangliomas
- **Incidence**: unknown in the US population. In the Dutch population, familial cases cause about 50% of all paraganglioma cases, corresponding to an incidence of approximately one in 1 million.
- **Inheritance pattern**: autosomal dominant. However, a unique parent-of-origin effect is consistently reported for hereditary paraganglioma (PGL) type 1: offspring of female gene carriers do not develop disease, whereas 50% of offspring of male gene carriers do. This observation is consistent with genomic imprinting of the associated gene, but no evidence of parentally determined methylation has been demonstrated for SDHD. No parent-of-origin effect is found for familial paraganglioma linked to the other susceptibility loci.
- **Gene and chromosomal location**: hereditary PGL1 is caused by mutations in SDHD, at 11q23. PGL2 maps to 11q13.1 and is caused by SDHAF2. PGL3 is caused by mutations in SDHC on 1q21. PGL4 is caused by mutations in SDHB at 1p36. PGL5 is caused by mutations in SDHA at 1q23.3. All these genes are required for structure and function of complex II of the respiratory chain (succinate-ubiquinone oxidoreductase, succinate dehydrogenase, SDH), that may regulate the response of the carotid body to hypoxia. Loss of function of these genes results in chronic hypoxic stimulation and cellular proliferation and/or neoplasia.
- **Mutations**: two founder mutations, Asp92Tyr and Leu139Pro, have been found in the SDHD gene. Various mutations have been found in SDHB and SDHC. In most cases, mutations lead to protein truncation. Mutations were mostly unique to each family.
- **Associated malignant neoplasms**: approximately 10% of hereditary paragangliomas undergo malignant degeneration. Patients with the SDHB mutation are more likely to develop malignant disease and intra-abdominal tumors. Patients with all SDH

mutations may also be at risk of other tumor types, including renal cell cancer (in SDHB), astrocytomas, papillary thyroid carcinoma, and parathyroid adenoma.
- **Associated benign neoplasms**: carotid body paragangliomas, which account for 78% of all head and neck paragangliomas discovered. Adrenal paragangliomas (pheochromocytomas) occur. C-cell hyperplasia now reported in a family with SDHD mutation.

Li–Fraumeni Syndrome (LFS) (Including Li-Fraumeni-Like Syndrome)

- **LFS** (Upton et al. 2009) is a disease associated with an increased risk of developing cancer.
- **Incidence**: LFS appears to be rare, with approximately 400 reported families in the cumulative literature, but its actual population incidence is unknown.
- **Inheritance pattern**: autosomal dominant. Penetrance is almost complete and appears to be gender-dependent, the lifetime risk of developing cancer being higher in women.
- **Gene and chromosomal location**: TP53, at 17p13.1. p53, the protein encoded by TP53, regulates the cell-cycle arrest that is required to permit repair of DNA damage. In p53 mutation-negative LFS families (most of which meet Li-Fraumeni-Like [LFL] criteria), germline CHEK2 mutations have been reported. CHEK2 (located at 22q12.1) is in the p53 pathway, and germline mutations were originally found in a few LFL families. Currently, there is disagreement as to whether CHEK2 truly causes LFS or LFL, or whether it is etiologically related only to the early-onset breast cancers which occur in this disorder. The CHEK2*1100delC mutation, the frequency of which varies across populations, appears to increase risk of breast cancer by about twofold and may predispose to earlier age at diagnosis. A third LFS locus has been mapped to chromosome 1q23, but no specific gene has yet been implicated.
- **Mutations**: when clinical mutation testing targets only exons 5–8, as is often done, approximately 70% of Li–Fraumeni families meeting the stringent diagnostic criteria have p53 mutations. Mutations in exons 4–9 are found in 95% of such families. LFL kindreds have detectable mutations in 8%–22% of probands, depending upon the stringency of the syndrome definition. Overall, about 75% of p53 mutations involve exons 5 through 8. Missense mutations represent the majority (approximately 75%) of genetic lesions, and most generate a truncated p53 protein. A web-based repository of p53 mutation information has been created (http://www-p53.iarc.fr/index.html); it contains information on nearly 300 deleterious germline mutations.
- **Associated malignant neoplasms**: risk of developing any invasive cancer (excluding skin cancer) was approximately 50% by age 30 (compared with 1% in the general population), and approximately 90% by age 70. The tumor spectrum includes osteogenic and chondrosarcoma, rhabdomyosarcoma, breast cancer, brain cancer (especially glioblastomas), leukemia, lymphoma, and adrenocortical carcinoma.

Early-onset breast cancer accounts for 25% of all LFS-related cancers, followed by soft-tissue sarcoma, bone sarcoma, and brain tumors. The risks of sarcoma, female breast cancer, and hematopoietic malignancies in mutation carriers are more than 100 times greater than those seen in the general population.

The "classical" LFS malignancies (sarcoma and cancers of the breast, brain, and adrenal glands) comprise about 80% of all cancers that occur in LFS families. The incidence of these cancers varies by age, with soft-tissue sarcomas, adrenal and brain tumors predominating before age 10, bone sarcoma the most frequent in the teen years, and breast and brain tumors comprising the majority after age 20. Relative to LFL families, kindreds meeting stringent LFS criteria have more brain tumors, earlier onset of breast cancer, and exclusive occurrence of adrenocortical carcinoma.

- **Associated benign neoplasms**: none known.

Multiple Endocrine Neoplasia Type 1 (MEN1)

- MEN (Rubinstein 2010) syndromes are associated to the development of benign or malignant tumors in the endocrine glands. Sometimes the glands grow too large but do have not tumors.
- **Incidence**: estimated to 1 in 50,000 people in general population.
- **Inheritance pattern**: Autosomal dominant. The age-related penetrance of MEN1 is 45% at age 30 years, 82% at age 50 years, and 96% at age 70 years.
- **Gene and chromosomal location**: MEN1 at 11q13. The functions of menin, the protein encoded by MEN1, are inferred from its interactions with other proteins, like JunD, NFκB and p53, among many others. Hence, it seems that menin plays a role in transcription regulation, cellular proliferation, apoptosis and genome stability.
- **Mutations**: more than 400 different frameshift, nonsense, missense, insertion, and deletion mutations have been reported. Ten percent of germline mutations are *de novo*. A trend toward overrepresentation of truncating mutations was observed among those developing thymic carcinoid tumors.
- **Associated malignant neoplasms**: pancreatic or duodenal neuroendocrine tumors occur in 30%–80% of patients with MEN1; pancreatic endocrine tumors are the most common cause of death. Gastrinomas, often multicentric, occur in 54% of mutation carriers and are most often in the duodenum (90% of gastrinomas) or head of pancreas. Malignant islet cell tumors (glucagonomas, VIPomas, PTHrPomas, insulinomas) are treated with resection. Insulinomas (benign or malignant) occur in less than 10% of MEN1 cases but are the most common functioning pancreatic endocrine tumor in MEN1 patients younger than age 25 years. Less than 10% of individuals with insulinomas have MEN1. Glucagonomas occur in approximately 3% of MEN1 patients. Carcinoids are the second most common cause of death in MEN1 and are more likely to arise in the thymus, bronchus, or stomach than are sporadic carcinoids. Up to 25% of thymic carcinoids are due to MEN1. Gastroduodenal carcinoids may be either nonfunctioning or secrete gastrin or serotonin products. Malignant schwannoma, ovarian tumors, pancreatic islet cell carcinomas,

adrenocortical carcinomas, non-medullary thyroid neoplasms, and gastrointestinal stromal tumor have also been reported in mutation carriers.
- **Associated benign neoplasms**: hyperparathyroidism (HPT) is present in more than 95% of MEN1 patients and occurs at younger ages than sporadic HPT, with hypercalcemia reported in 66%, 85%, and 87% of MEN1 patients by ages 25, 55, or older, respectively. Anterior pituitary adenomas are found in 10%–60% of patients with MEN1 (of which two-thirds are prolactinomas); note that about 10% of the general population have microadenomas. Pituitary adenomas may secrete ACTH (about 5%), growth hormone (about 25%), or be nonsecretory (about 10%) and tend to be larger, more aggressive tumors than their sporadic counterparts. Adrenal cortical adenomas are said to occur in 35% of individuals with MEN1. Most are nonfunctioning but they may produce aldosterone or cortisol (Cushing syndrome). Multiple lipomas (30%), collagenomas (5%), tumors secreting vasointestinal peptide, thyroid neoplasms (non-medullary thyroid cancer), facial angiofibromas (75%, usually on the lip or other area not generally seen in tuberous sclerosis), meningiomas (5%), ependymomas (1%), and leiomyomas (10%) have also been reported.

Multiple Endocrine Neoplasia Type 2A, 2B (MEN2)

- **MEN** syndromes (Rubinstein 2010) are associated to the development of benign or malignant tumors in the endocrine glands. Sometimes the glands grow too large but do have not tumors.
- **Incidence**: one in 30,000 births. About 3–10% of all thyroid cancers are medullary thyroid cancer (MTC).
- **Inheritance pattern**: autosomal dominant.
- **Gene and chromosomal location**: RET, at 10q11.2.
- **Mutations**: RET mutations are identifiable in more than 98% of cases of multiple endocrine neoplasia type 2A (MEN2A) and 85% of familial medullary thyroid cancer (FMTC), in which they involve exons 10 and 11, targeting one of five cysteines in the extracellular binding domain of the encoded protein. MEN2B is characterized by a M918T mutation in codon 918 of exon 16 in 95% of cases and an A883F mutation in exon 15 in most of the others. Nearly all germline RET mutations causing MEN2A and FMTC are inherited; 40% of mutations causing MEN2B occur *de novo*. Mutations associated with MEN2A are reported to accelerate cell proliferation, whereas those associated with MEN2B enhance suppression of apoptosis. These differential effects are hypothesized to account for some of the clinical differences between these groups of patients.
- **Associated malignant neoplasms**: medullary thyroid cancer (MTC) with metastatic disease reported as early as ages 3 and 5 in MEN2B and MEN2A, respectively. Pheochromocytomas are malignant in 10% and are bilateral (either synchronous or metachronous) in one-third of patients. MTC is almost always diagnosed before the age of 40 in MEN2A and MEN2B. MTC in FMTC is a more indolent disease, with

onset often after the age of 50 years. Papillary thyroid cancer has also been associated with MEN 2 and FMTC.
- **Associated benign neoplasms**: hyperparathyroidism (HPT) is found in 10%–20% of individuals with MEN2A; however, this condition is rare in MEN2B. Pheochromocytomas are most often benign. Ganglioneuromas of the gastrointestinal tract and mucosal neuromas are present in nearly all patients with MEN2B.

MYH-Associated Polyposis (MAP)

- **MAP** (Goodenberger and Lindor 2011) is a disease associated with the development of multiple (between 15 and 100) adenomatous colon polyps and an increased risk of colorectal cancer. Patients test negative for a mutation in APC (such mutations are related to Familial Adenomatous Polyposis (FAP)).
- **Incidence**: in the general population, approximately 1% are heterozygous (monoallelic) MYH mutation carriers. In large population-based series of colorectal cancer cases, biallelic MYH mutations were found in 0.54%–1%.
- **Inheritance pattern**: autosomal recessive.
- **Gene and chromosomal location**: MYH (MUTYH) on 1p32.1–p34.3. It encodes a base-excision repair gene, the product of which participates in repair of mutations caused by reactive oxygen species.
- **Mutations**: North American studies suggest that two mutations (Y165C and G382D) account for 80%–85% of mutations occurring in individuals of Caucasian ancestry; early evidence suggests that the Y165C mutation may be more deleterious. If only these mutations are tested, true biallelic carriers would have both mutations identified in approximately 72% of cases, only one mutation identified in approximately 26% of cases, and no mutation detected in approximately 2%.
- **Associated malignant neoplasms**: excess risks of colon cancer and duodenal cancer occur in biallelic MYH mutation carriers.
- **Associated benign neoplasms**: colonic and duodenal adenomas; gastric fundic gland polyps; osteomas, sebaceous gland adenomas, pilomatricomas (suggestive of Muir–Torre syndrome variant of Lynch syndrome).

Neurofibromatosis Type 1 (NF1)

- **NF1** (DiGiovanna and Kraemer 2010) is a condition commonly associated with multiple café-au-lait spots on the skin and the development of varying numbers of neurofibromas
- **Incidence**: One in 3000; one-third to one-half of cases represents a new germline mutation.
- **Inheritance pattern**: autosomal dominant. High penetrance.
- **Gene and chromosomal location**: NF1 at 17q11.2; encodes a Ras guanosine triphosphate–activating protein known as neurofibromin. Recent studies suggest that

neurofibromin plays a role in the adenylate cyclase and AKT-mTOR signaling pathways and modulates cell motility by binding with actin in the cytoskeleton.
- **Mutations**: unique from family to family; all types of mutations have been reported. No genotype–phenotype correlations have been established except for those with deletions of the whole gene, which is associated with facial dysmorphism, early onset of neurofibromas, a higher frequency of learning disabilities, and malignant peripheral nerve sheath tumors (MPNSTs), and a 3 basepair deletion in exon 17 associated with only cutaneous pigmentary features.
- **Associated malignant neoplasms**: MPNSTs, formerly called neurofibrosarcomas or malignant schwannomas, occur in 3%–15% of affected individuals and typically develop in preexisting plexiform neurofibromas. Conversely, it has been estimated that 50% of individuals with MPNSTs have NF1. Outcome appears to be worse for NF1-associated MPNSTs compared with sporadic MPNSTs. Also, there is increased risk (no greater than 1%) for astrocytomas, carcinoids (usually duodenal), pheochromocytomas, neuroblastomas, ependymomas, primitive neuroectodermal tumors, rhabdomyosarcomas (especially of the pelvis), and undifferentiated sarcomas as well as for Wilms tumor and leukemia (juvenile myelomonocytic leukemia). About 15% of children with NF1 have signs of optic pathway tumors by imaging studies, due to pilocytic astrocytoma. Malignant optic nerve gliomas also occur, causing vision loss and other neurological symptoms due to direct extension into the brain.
- **Associated benign neoplasms**: peripheral, nodular, or plexiform neurofibromas; benign pheochromocytomas, meningiomas; Lisch nodules of the iris; and hamartomatous intestinal polyps. Gastrointestinal stromal tumors (preferentially of the small intestine) can arise via hyperplasia of the interstitial cells of Cajal, located within the intestinal wall. Although some optic nerve gliomas are histologically benign, they are still a source of marked clinical morbidity.

Neurofibromatosis Type 2 (NF2)

- **NF2** (DiGiovanna and Kraemer 2010) is a condition most commonly associated with bilateral vestibular schwannomas. There is also an increased risk of other tumors of the nervous system.
- **Incidence**: one in 35 000, of which 50% have de novo mutations. About 7% of vestibular schwannomas are due to NF2.
- **Inheritance pattern**: autosomal dominant.
- **Gene and chromosomal location**: Neurofibromatosis type 2 (NF2) at 22q12.2. It encodes a protein designated neurofibromin-2 (also called merlin). It functions as a tumor suppressor and a regulator of Schwann cell and leptomeningeal cell proliferation.
- **Mutations**: More than 150 mutations (none are common) have been reported in NF2. Nonsense or frameshift mutations are associated with younger age at onset of symptoms and a greater number of tumors. Approximately 25% of individuals with *de novo* gene mutations are mosaic for the mutation, increasing the difficulty of

making a molecular diagnosis. Chromosomal changes detectable on karyotyping are infrequent. Large submicroscopic deletions encompassing the NF2 gene affect 10% of families and are not associated with cognitive impairment even if quite large. Cytogenetically visible deletions do cause cognitive impairment and/or congenital anomalies. Ring chromosome 22 has been reported in patients with multiple meningiomas and vestibular schwannomas fulfilling NF2 criteria. Apparently the ring contains the NF2 locus, but the ring may be lost somatically.

- **Associated malignant neoplasms**: gliomas (4%), ependymomas (3%). Astrocytomas and ependymomas may present as intramedullary tumors in approximately one-third of NF2 patients with spinal cord tumor.
- **Associated benign neoplasms**: vestibular schwannomas (acoustic neuromas), meningiomas, and spinal cord schwannomas (in about two-thirds subjects). Individuals who develop a unilateral vestibular schwannoma younger than age 30 are at high risk of having NF2, whereas those who develop unilateral disease older than age 55 seldom have NF2. Two-thirds of patients with NF2 develop intramedullary spinal cord tumors, usually multiple, although not always symptomatic. Most often these are schwannomas, which present a "dumbbell shape" on imaging studies, as the tumor extends medially and laterally through the foramina. Approximately 50% of patients with NF2 develop intracranial or spinal meningiomas.

Nijmegen Breakage Syndrome (NBS)

- **NBS** (Antoccia et al. 2006) is a disorder characterized by microcephaly, a distinct facial appearance, short stature, immunodeficiency, radiation sensitivity, and a strong predisposition to lymphoid malignancy.
- **Incidence**: NBS is most common in East European/Slavic population, where the carrier rate is closer to one in 100. In Germany, the carrier rate is one in 866 and one in 3 million is affected with NBS.
- **Inheritance pattern**: Autosomal recessive.
- **Gene and chromosomal location**: NBS1 at 8q21 encodes a protein designated nibrin. Like the ATM gene product, nibrin is involved in DNA double-strand break repair.
- **Mutations**: most are truncating mutations. In the United States, 70% of NBS patients are homozygous for one common founder mutation (657del5) and 15% are compound heterozygotes (having two different mutant alleles).
- **Associated malignant neoplasms**: about 35% of patients (70 reported cases) develop a malignancy, typically before age 15 years, most often a B-cell lymphoma or other hematopoietic malignancy. Patients with lower levels of intracellular nibrin appear to be at greater risk of lymphoma. Glioma, rhabdomyosarcoma, and medulloblastoma have been reported. NBS1 mutation carriers may be at increased risk of breast cancer, gastrointestinal lymphoma, and gastric and colorectal cancers.
- **Associated benign neoplasms**: none reported.

Peutz–Jeghers Syndrome (PJS)

- **PJS** (Beggs et al. 2010) is a disorder characterized by intestinal hamartomatous polyps in association with a distinct pattern of skin and mucosal macular melanin deposition. Patients with PJS have a 15-fold increased risk of developing intestinal cancer compared with that of the general population.
- **Incidence**: approximately 1 in 200,000 people.
- **Inheritance pattern**: autosomal dominant. Nearly complete penetrance.
- **Gene and chromosomal location**: STK11 (previously LKB1) at 19p13.3. It encodes a master kinase targeting the family of AMP-activated kinases (AMPKs). Through activation of multiple signaling pathways, LKB1's main physiologic functions involve regulating cellular growth, metabolism, and polarity. Some studies suggest locus heterogeneity.
- **Mutations**: STK11 mutations have been found in 70% of individuals with a positive family history of Peutz–Jeghers Syndrome (PJS) and in 20%–70% of individuals with clinical PJS, without affected relatives. Mutations are presumed deleterious due to loss of function. Sixteen to forty percent of mutations involve large gene deletions.
- **Associated malignant neoplasms**: gastrointestinal cancers as a group are the most common malignancies in PJS patients. Cumulative risks from age 15 to 64 is 93% for all cancers combined and 0.5% esophagus, 29% stomach, 13% small intestine, 39% colon, 36% pancreas, 15% lung, 9% testes, 54% breast, 9% uterus, 21% ovary, and 10% cervix.
- **Associated benign neoplasms**: multiple PJS polyps occur throughout the gastrointestinal tract, most commonly the jejunum, ileum, and duodenum. Polyps occasionally occur in the nose, bronchi, renal pelvis, ureters, and bladder. Age at onset of symptoms is variable, sometimes developing in the first years of life. Ovarian tumors in affected individuals are "sex cord tumors with annular tubules," which are considered characteristic of PJS, and are present in almost all affected females. Males may develop Sertoli cell tumors of the testis.

Polyposis, Familial Juvenile (FJP)

- **FJP** (Brosens et al. 2011) is a disorder characterized by predisposition to hamartomatous polyps in the gastrointestinal tract, specifically in the stomach, small intestine, colon, and rectum.
- **Incidence**: estimated between one in 16,000 and one in 100,000 live births. In all, 20%–50% of all FJP cases are inherited.
- **Inheritance pattern**: autosomal dominant.
- **Gene and chromosomal location**: BMPR1A at 10q and SMAD4 at 18q21.1 account for approximately 25% and 15%–20% of FJP, respectively. Some cases of FJP were ascribed to PTEN mutations at 10q22.3; it is currently thought that other features of PTEN hamartoma tumor syndrome and/or Cowden syndrome distinguish these cases from true FJP.

- **Mutations**: most mutations in the causative genes result in truncated proteins, predicting a tumor suppressor gene function. Increased prevalence of massive gastric polyposis was reported in patients with SMAD4 mutations compared with BMPR1A mutation patients.
- **Associated malignant neoplasms**: risk estimates for developing gastrointestinal malignancy range from 9% to 68% and vary with the gene involved. Colorectal cancer accounts for most of the excess cancer risk in FJP. In one kindred with a SMAD4 mutation, the lifetime risks of colorectal and other gastrointestinal cancer (stomach, duodenal, pancreatic) were 40% and 20%, respectively.
- **Associated benign neoplasms**: gastrointestinal polyps involving the stomach (which can be very extensive), small bowel, and colorectum. Colorectal adenoma has also been reported.

Retinoblastoma (RB), Hereditary

- **Retinoblastoma** (Aerts et al. 2006), which is usually found in infants and toddlers, is cancer of the eye. It first arises in the retina, but can move to other parts of the body.
- **Incidence**: retinoblastoma has an incidence of one in 13,500 to one in 25,000 live births. Approximately 60% are unilateral and nonhereditary, 15% are unilateral and hereditary, and 25% are bilateral and hereditary. Males and females are equally affected. Approximately 20%– 30% of mutation-positive individuals have de novo mutations. The frequency of gene mutation carriers in the general population is unknown.
- **Inheritance pattern**: autosomal dominant with incomplete penetrance (estimated at 90%).
- **Gene and chromosomal location**: RB1 at 13q14. It encodes a tumor suppressor gene that regulates cell cycle progression and cellular differentiation.
- **Mutations**: many distinct deletions (large and small) and point mutations distributed widely across RB1 have been reported. The majority of classical families show nonsense and frameshift mutations. Lower penetrance RB families have in-frame deletions, missense mutations, and mutations in the promoter region. In bilateral RB patients, splice-site mutations are associated with late age at RB onset. Chromosomal deletions of 13q14 have been reported in a minority of individuals with RB: 5% in unilateral RB and 7.5% with bilateral RB. Deletions are also found as a somatic mosaic abnormality in some affected individuals.
- **Associated malignant neoplasms**: family members with an affected parent and sibling have a 900-fold increase in RB risk. Second malignant tumors in RB patients were originally attributed exclusively to the carcinogenic effects of therapeutic irradiation; radiation treatment increases the risk of second cancers by threefold. However, it is now clear that some second cancers occur without prior radiation exposure. Approximately 1% of patients with bilateral (hereditary) RB develop a nonocular second primary tumor (SPT) each year; at least 50% die of these second malignant neoplasms. For those who survive an SPT, there is approximately 2% per year risk of developing a third tumor. Osteosarcoma is the most common second

tumor (500-fold risk increase) in RB patients. Melanoma, brain tumors, and nasal cavity cancers also occur excessively. Fibrosarcomas, chondrosarcomas, rhabdomyosarcomas, Ewing's sarcomas, leukemias, lymphomas, pinealoblastomas, and malignant phyllodes tumors have also been reported. It has been reported a statistically elevated 15-fold risk of death from lung cancer among patients with hereditary RB. Carriers of RB1 mutations appear be highly-susceptible to smoking-induced lung cancers.
- **Associated benign neoplasms**: retinomas, benign retinal tumors, and lipomas.

Rhabdoid Tumor Predisposition Syndrome (RTPS)

- **RTPS** (Teplick et al. 2011) is a disease characterized by a marked predisposition toward the development of malignant rhabdoid tumors of infancy and early childhood. The atypical teratoid/rhabdoid tumor (AT/RT) is by far the most common CNS malignancy associated with this syndrome.
- **Incidence**: extremely rare.
- **Inheritance pattern**: autosomal dominant, with incomplete penetrance.
- **Gene and chromosomal location**: SMARCB1 at 22q11.2. It encodes a core member of the SWI/SNF chromatin remodeling complex, which regulate local chromatin structure and is a critical component of the mechanisms for controlling gene expression. The existence of a second susceptibility gene is indicated by an extensively characterized family not linked to SMARCB1.
- **Mutations**: a variety of biallelic somatic mutations and deletions have been found in SMARCB1. Germline SMARCB1 mutations have been identified in a subset of families with malignant RTs and various central nervous system neoplasms.
- **Associated malignant neoplasms**: renal and extrarenal malignant AT/RTs, choroid plexus carcinoma, medulloblastoma, and central PNET have also been reported.
- **Associated benign neoplasms**: meningioma, myoepithelioma and familial schwannomatosis.

Rothmund–Thomson Syndrome (RTS)

- **RTS** (Monnat 2010) is a genodermatosis presenting with a characteristic facial rash (poikiloderma) associated with short stature, sparse scalp hair, sparse or absent eyelashes and/or eyebrows, juvenile cataracts, skeletal abnormalities, radial ray defects, premature aging and a predisposition to cancer.
- **Incidence**: very rare. Approximately 300 cases of RTS have been reported in the scientific literature.
- **Inheritance pattern**: autosomal recessive.
- **Gene and chromosomal location**: RECQL4 gene on chromosome 8q24.3. It encodes a helicase, a protein that binds to DNA and temporarily unwinds its double helix structure, thus allowing DNA replication in preparation for cell division and for repairing damaged DNA. Rothmund–Thomson syndrome (RTS) is a member of the

RecQ helicase chromosomal instability disorders, which also include Bloom and Werner syndromes.
- **Mutations**: to date, more than 25 different mutations have been described in RECQL4
- **Associated malignant neoplasms**: osteosarcoma, non-melanoma skin malignancies: squamous cell carcinomas, Bowen's diseases, basal cell carcinoma, spindle cell carcinoma. Cancer of the tongue, acute myeloblastic leukemia, progressive leukopenia, myelodysplasia and aplastic anemia have also been reported. Because of the very small number of RTS patients, it is unclear which, if any, of these associations are significant; risks of specific sites or types of cancers have not yet been defined, except for osteogenic sarcoma.
- **Associated benign neoplasms**: warty dyskeratosis, actinic keratoses.

Shwachman-Bodian-Diamond Syndrome (SBDS)

- **SBDS** (Burroughs et al. 2009) is a disorder characterized by exocrine pancreatic insufficiency, bone marrow dysfunction, skeletal abnormalities, and short stature.
- **Incidence**: estimated to 1 in 50,000 births, but there is no scientific basis for this number because there is no simple way of establishing the diagnosis
- **Inheritance**: autosomal recessive
- **Gene and location**: SBDS, at 7q11.21. It encodes a protein involved in ribosome biogenesis.
- **Mutations**: several mutations have been identified but the two most common mutations are the consequence of 183–184 TA>CT and 258+2T>C genomic changes. These mutations are located in exon 2 and intron 2, and result in a premature stop-codon (K62X) and a frameshift mutation resulting in a stopcodon (C84fsX3) respectively.
- **Associated malignant neoplasms**: the risk for AML in SDS is estimated to be 15-25%. MDS has been found in small cohorts of SDS patients in 10-44%. The predilection to malignant myeloid transformation is higher in SDS patients with evolving pancytopenia and can already occur during infancy.
- **Associated benign neoplasms**: none reported.

Simpson–Golabi–Behmel Syndrome (SGBS)

- **SGBS** (Sabin et al. 2011) is a condition associated with general overgrowth in height and weight. Individuals with SGBS also have characteristic facial features in childhood.
- **Incidence**: unknown. Approximately 100 patients had been reported by 1999.
- **Inheritance pattern**: X-linked recessive (mild manifestations in carrier females).
- **Gene and chromosomal location**: SGBS type 1 (SGBS1) is caused by mutations in GPC3 (at Xq26), the glypican-3 gene, an extracellular glycoprotein thought to have a role in control of embryonic mesoderm. SGBS2 is caused by mutations in OFD1 (at

Xp22) and is allelic with orofacial digital syndrome type I. OFD1 encodes a component of the distal centriole that controls centriole length
- **Mutations**: inactivating mutations in GPC3 are reported (including large and small deletions of different exons, splice sites, and point mutations) with neither mutational hotspots nor genotype–phenotype correlations appreciated to date. An OFD1 mutation in a single family with a very severe phenotype was reported. The exact role of GPC3 in the etiology of SGBS is still unknown.
- **Associated malignant neoplasms** SGBS patients have an increased risk of embryonal malignancies, especially Wilms tumor. Neuroblastomas, hepatoblastoma, hepatocellular carcinoma, and testicular gonadoblastoma have also been reported.
- **Associated benign neoplasms**: none reported.

Tuberous Sclerosis Complex (TSC)

- **TSC** (Tomasoni and Mondino 2011) is a disorder associated to tumors in many different organs, primarily in the brain, eyes, heart, kidney, skin and lungs.
- **Incidence**: TSC is estimated to be present in one of 5,800 live births. Prevalence is approximately one in 30,000 individuals younger than age of 65 and approximately one in 15,000 younger than age of 5.
- **Inheritance pattern**: autosomal dominant.
- **Gene and chromosomal location**: TSC1 on 9q34; TSC2 on 16p13.3. Their protein products are designated hamartin and tuberin, respectively. Mutations in one or the other of these genes are detectable in about 80% of individuals with tuberous sclerosis complex (TSC), with higher detection rates for TSC2 than TSC1, despite linkage studies suggesting similar prevalence of these two genes.
- **Mutations**: TSC1 mutations tend to be small deletions, insertions, or nonsense mutations, whereas TSC2 mutations tend to be large deletions and rearrangements (which cannot be detected by sequencing). More than 60% of cases represent de novo mutations. Between 10% and 25% of patients show somatic mosaicism, which presents a milder phenotype. The TSC2 and PKD1 genes are located next to one another in opposite orientation. A large deletion of the 3' end of either gene may affect the function of both genes, leading to a contiguous gene syndrome of severe autosomal dominant polycystic kidney disease in infancy.
- **Associated malignant neoplasms**: there is a 6%–14% incidence of childhood brain tumors in patients with TSC, of which more than 90% are subependymal giant cell astrocytomas. TSC is associated with a cumulative renal cancer incidence of 2.2%–4.4%. The renal abnormalities in TSC are unusual in that patients develop epithelial lesions (cysts; oncocytomas; and clear cell, papillary, or chromophobe carcinomas) as well as mesenchymal lesions (angiomyolipomas), suggesting that the TSC genes regulate early differentiation and proliferation of renal precursor cells. Malignant angiomyolipoma is reported in less than 1% of individuals with TSC. Wilms tumor, Hurthle cell thyroid cancer, and chordoma have been reported in TSC families, but whether these are true associations is unknown.

- **Associated benign neoplasms**: cortical and subcortical tubers (glial harmartomas) (70%), subependymal glial nodules (90%), retinal hamartomas or achromic patches (75%).

Variegated Aneuploidy, Mosaic (MVA)

- MVA (García-Castillo et al. 2008) is a disorder characterized by growth retardation of prenatal onset, microcephaly, developmental delay, structural central nervous system, ophthalmological anomalies, and mild dysmorphic features
- **Incidence**: rare.
- **Inheritance pattern**: autosomal recessive.
- **Gene and chromosomal location**: BUB1B at 15q15. It encodes a protein involved in mitotic spindle checkpoint regulation.
- **Mutations**: may be either missense or truncating.
- **Associated malignant neoplasms**: embryonal rhabdomyosarcoma seems most strongly associated, with Wilms tumor and leukemias also reported.
- **Associated benign neoplasms**: none known.

Von Hippel–Lindau Syndrome (VHL)

- VHL (Maher et al. 2011) is a multisystem disorder characterized by abnormal growth of blood vessels resulting in hemangioblastomas and cysts, as well as development of other tumors in multiple organs.
- **Incidence**: approximately one in 30,000–40,000.
- **Inheritance pattern**: autosomal dominant. The penetrance is age-dependent, but reaches 95–100% by age 65.
- **Gene and chromosomal location**: VHL on 3p25–p26. VHL has been implicated in a variety of cellular functions including extracellular matrix formation and cell cycle exit. Perhaps its most well-characterized role is the regulation of hypoxia-inducible factor 1 (HIF1). HIF1 is a heterodimer (with a- and b-subunits), which in hypoxic conditions binds DNA and activates transcription of a number of downstream genes that are involved in energy metabolism, angiogenesis, and apoptosis.
- **Mutations**: more than 300 different pathogenic DNA variants have been reported; 72% are missense mutations, and 28% are partial or complete gene deletions. Germline VHL mutations can be detected in nearly 100% of clinically affected individuals. Families may be characterized by the presence (VHL type 2: 7%–20% of families) or absence (VHL type 1) of pheochromocytomas. Approximately 95% of type 2 families have missense mutations, whereas approximately 96% of type 1 families have deletions or premature termination mutations.
- **Associated malignant neoplasms**: Von Hippel-Lindau is a devastating cancer syndrome, predisposing to various types of cancer: malignant renal cell carcinoma (RCC; clear cell type) occurs in 35%–75% of affected individuals in autopsy series and in 25%–38% in clinical series. Pancreatic islet cell carcinomas tend to cluster in

certain families, in which the incidence ranges from 7.5% to 25%. Carcinoid tumors have been reported occasionally. Pheochromocytomas rarely undergo malignant transformation. Endolymphatic sac tumors are locally aggressive papillary adenocarcinomas. They have been reported in 11%–16% of VHL patients, and in 14%–30%, they are bilateral; they cause hearing loss, tinnitus, and vertigo.
- **Associated benign neoplasms**: hemangioblastomas, which are histologically benign tumors, occur in 50%–79% of autopsy-confirmed cases and in 18%–44% of patients in clinical series; they are the cause of the first VHL symptoms in 40% of patients and cause more than 50% of the deaths. Retinal angiomas (which are also hemangioblastomas) occur in approximately 70% of individuals and can result in visual loss. Pancreatic cystadenomas are found in 7% of patients. Pancreatic cystadenoma is a benign nonfunctional tumor that should be differentiated from a pancreatic islet cell carcinoma. A total of 20%–100% of patients have renal lesions. Cystic lesions are by far the most common, and complex cysts can contain RCC. Pheochromocytoma occurs in 3.5%–17% of VHL patients and tends to cluster in certain kindreds; 26%–34% of these lesions are bilateral. Epididymal cysts are found in 7%–27% of patients, ranging in size from 0.5–2.0 cm. Benign epididymal papillary cystadenomas are found in 3%–26% of males on autopsy series. The equivalent lesion reported in women is papillary cystadenoma of the broad ligament. Hepatic cysts (in 17% of patients) have been reported in autopsy series. Splenic angiomas and cysts occur in 3%–7% of autopsied patients.

Werner Syndrome (WS)

- **WS** (Ozgenc and Loeb 2006) is a syndrome characterized by the dramatic, rapid appearance of features associated with normal aging.
- **Incidence**: Estimated at one in 50,000 to one in 1,000,000 live births.
- **Inheritance pattern**: autosomal recessive.
- **Gene and chromosomal location**: WRN (8p11.2–p12) encodes a DNA helicase of the RecQ family involved with DNA recombination, replication, and repair. Mutations in other members of the RecQ family are causative of Rothmund–Thomson syndrome and Bloom syndrome, providing a hypothesis for the phenotypic similarities among these disorders.
- **Mutations**: Multiple unique mutations have been identified; nearly all lead to premature protein truncation. One founder mutation accounts for 60% of mutations in Japan.
- **Associated malignant neoplasms**: soft-tissue sarcomas, melanomas (which occurred in unusual locations, especially intranasally and on the soles of the feet), osteosarcomas, hematologic malignancies, epithelial cancers (thyroid, gastric, breast, hepatocellular, biliary).
- **Associated benign neoplasms** RAEB[t]: meningiomas.

Wilms Tumor, Familial

- **WT** (Hamilton and Shamberger 2012) is a disorder characterized by kidney cancer in children. It causes a tumor on one or both kidneys.
- **Incidence**: one in 10,000 general population live births. WT accounts for more than 90% of childhood renal tumors, with a median age of onset of 3–4 years and declining rapidly thereafter. Ninety-five percent of WT occur as a sporadic event in children with no recognizable syndromic findings. In this group, it is unclear how many are truly sporadic tumors vs. the number having new (de novo) mutations or inherited predisposition of a gene of low penetrance. Only 1%–2% of patients with WT have a family history of WT.
- **Inheritance pattern**: autosomal dominant.
- **Gene and chromosomal location**: familial Wilms tumor (FWT) is genetically heterogeneous. The WT1 gene (11p13) is the only gene identified that causes a nonsyndromic FWT. It accounts however for only a minority of FWT. FWT1 (WT4), FWT2, WT3, and WT5, located on chromosomes 17q12–q21, 19q, 16q, and 7p11.2–p15, respectively, are additional loci for which linkage to FWT has been reported, but specific genes have not yet been cloned. The 11p15 locus (associated with Beckwith–Weidemann syndrome [BWS]) is often referred to as WT2, although the gene at this locus has yet to be identified.
- **Mutations**: while fewer than 5% of apparently sporadic Wilms tumors have germline WT1 mutations, those that do have earlier age at diagnosis (approximately age 1 vs. age 4) and are more likely to be bilateral (38% vs. 5%). Mutations in WT1 are also associated with several syndromes whose risk of Wilms tumor is estimated as greater than 20% [reviewed by Scott et al. (2)]. The Denys–Drash Syndrome (DDS; triad of Wilms tumor, nephropathy, and genitourinary tract anomalies including possible pseudohermaphrodism in males) is associated with an intragenic WT1 mutation in 90%. Selected point mutations in the zinc-finger domains of WT1 that affect the DNA-binding domains have a dominant-negative effect. The essential sclerosis of the kidney in DDS may lead to renal failure in early childhood.

    WAGR syndrome (Wilma tumor–anorexia–genitourinary–mental retardation) is found in approximately seven to eight per 1000 individuals with WT. Forty percent develop renal failure by age 20. Heterozygous micro deletion of 11p13 (encompassing WT1 and PAX6) results in Wilma tumor–anorexia syndrome, in which the PAX6 gene deletion explains the anorexia. About 30% of individuals with anorexia have deletions that include WT1. Larger deletions of this region account for the full WAGR phenotype. Frasier syndrome consists of nephropathy, gonad digenesis (including sex reversal in XY individuals), and gonadoblastoma. This is due to a splice site mutation in intron 9 of WT1, but does not include an increased risk of WT.
- **Associated malignant neoplasms**: Wilms tumor in the case of WT1 mutations.
- **Associated benign neoplasms**: nephrogenic rests.

Xeroderma Pigmentosum (Includes Complementation Groups A–G and XP Variant)

- **XP** (DiGiovanna and Kraemer 2012) is a condition characterized by an extreme sensitivity to ultraviolet rays from sunlight. This condition mostly affects the eyes and areas of skin exposed to the sun. Some affected individuals also have problems involving the nervous system
- **Incidence**: Approximately one in 1,000,000 live births in the United States, one in 40,000 in Japan (higher rates are observed in populations in which consanguinity is more prevalent).
- **Inheritance pattern**: autosomal recessive.
- **Genes and chromosomal locations**: See XP genes in chapter 1. Xeroderma pigmentosum (XP) genes A through G are involved in nucleotide excision repair (NER). In XP variant, the molecular basis is an error-prone DNA polymerase, which continues replication of damaged DNA by bypassing UV-induced thymidine dimers.
- **Mutations**: a variety of mutations have been reported in each of the cloned genes, usually point mutations.
- **Associated malignant neoplasms**: there is a 1,000-fold increased frequency of early-onset basal cell or squamous cell carcinomas and melanomas of the skin, often with multiple primary tumors, by age 20. The median age at first skin neoplasm diagnosis is 8 years, nearly 50 years younger than that found in the general population. A 5% risk of malignant melanoma is reported. Occasional sarcomas are observed. Ocular melanomas have been reported. The incidence of squamous cell carcinoma of the sunexposed tip of the tongue is increased 10,000-fold. A 10- to 20-fold increased risk of internal neoplasms has been reported, including brain tumors, cancers of the lung, uterus, breast, stomach, kidney, testicle, and leukemias. It is uncertain which of these cancers are truly manifestations of the XP syndrome. These cancers could theoretically result from unrepaired DNA damage caused by environmental carcinogens, such as those in tobacco smoke, or from endogenous metabolic oxidative DNA damage.
- **Associated benign neoplasms**: conjunctival papillomas, actinic keratoses, lid epitheliomas, keratoacanthomas, angiomas, and fibromas.

References

Aerts I, Lumbroso-Le Rouic L, Gauthier-Villars M, Brisse H, Doz F, Desjardins L. Retinoblastoma. *Orphanet J Rare Dis.* 2006 Aug 25;1:31.

Antoccia A, Kobayashi J, Tauchi H, Matsuura S, Komatsu K. Nijmegen breakage syndrome and functions of the responsible protein, NBS1. *Genome Dyn.* 2006;1:191-205.

Backes FJ, Cohn DE. Lynch syndrome. *Clin Obstet Gynecol.* 2011 Jun;54(2):199-214.

Basu B, Yap TA, Molife LR, de Bono JS. Targeting the DNA damage response in oncology: past, present and future perspectives. *Curr Opin Oncol.* 2012 May;24(3):316-24.

Beggs AD, Latchford AR, Vasen HF, Moslein G, Alonso A, Aretz S, Bertario L, Blanco I, Bülow S, Burn J, Capella G, Colas C, Friedl W, Møller P, Hes FJ, Järvinen H, Mecklin JP, Nagengast FM, Parc Y, Phillips RK, Hyer W, Ponz de Leon M, Renkonen-Sinisalo L, Sampson JR, Stormorken A, Tejpar S, Thomas HJ, Wijnen JT, Clark SK, Hodgson SV. Peutz-Jeghers syndrome: a systematic review and recommendations for management. *Gut.* 2010 Jul;59(7):975-86.

Brosens LA, Langeveld D, van Hattem WA, Giardiello FM, Offerhaus GJ. Juvenile polyposis syndrome. *World J Gastroenterol.* 2011 Nov 28;17(44):4839-44.

Burroughs L, Woolfrey A, Shimamura A. Shwachman-Diamond syndrome: a review of the clinical presentation, molecular pathogenesis, diagnosis, and treatment. *Hematol Oncol Clin North Am.* 2009 Apr;23(2):233-48.

Choufani S, Shuman C, Weksberg R. Beckwith-Wiedemann syndrome. *Am J Med Genet C Semin Med Genet.* 2010 Aug 15;154C(3):343-54.

DiGiovanna JJ, Kraemer KH. Shining a light on xeroderma pigmentosum. *J Invest Dermatol.* 2012 Mar;132(3 Pt 2):785-96. doi: 10.1038/jid.2011.426.

Ferner RE. The neurofibromatoses. *Pract Neurol.* 2010 Apr;10(2):82-93.

García-Castillo H, Vásquez-Velásquez AI, Rivera H, Barros-Núñez P. Clinical and genetic heterogeneity in patients with mosaic variegated aneuploidy: delineation of clinical subtypes. *Am J Med Genet A.* 2008 Jul 1;146A(13):1687-95.

Goodenberger M, Lindor NM. Lynch syndrome and MYH-associated polyposis: review and testing strategy. *J Clin Gastroenterol.* 2011 Jul;45(6):488-500.

Half E, Bercovich D, Rozen P. Familial adenomatous polyposis. *Orphanet J Rare Dis.* 2009 Oct 12;4:22.

Hamilton TE, Shamberger RC. Wilms tumor: recent advances in clinical care and biology. *Semin Pediatr Surg.* 2012 Feb;21(1):15-20

Jennes I, Pedrini E, Zuntini M, Mordenti M, Balkassmi S, Asteggiano CG, Casey B, Bakker B, Sangiorgi L, Wuyts W. Multiple osteochondromas: mutation update and description of the multiple osteochondromas mutation database (MOdb). *Hum Mutat.* 2009 Dec;30(12):1620-7.

Lacroix M, Leclercq G. The "portrait" of hereditary breast cancer. *Breast Cancer Res Treat.* 2005 Feb;89(3):297-304.

Lo Muzio L. Nevoid basal cell carcinoma syndrome (Gorlin syndrome). *Orphanet J Rare Dis.* 2008 Nov 25;3:32.

Maher ER, Neumann HP, Richard S. von Hippel-Lindau disease: a clinical and scientific review. *Eur J Hum Genet.* 2011 Jun;19(6):617-23

Maher ER. Genetics of familial renal cancers. *Nephron Exp Nephrol.* 2011;118(1):e21-6.

Marshall M, Solomon S. Hereditary breast-ovarian cancer: clinical findings and medical management. *Plast Surg Nurs.* 2007 Jul-Sep;27(3):124-7.

Mason PJ, Bessler M. The genetics of dyskeratosis congenita. *Cancer Genet.* 2011 Dec;204(12):635-45.

Monnat RJ Jr. Human RECQ helicases: roles in DNA metabolism, mutagenesis and cancer biology. *Semin Cancer Biol.* 2010 Oct;20(5):329-39.

Müller U. Pathological mechanisms and parent-of-origin effects in hereditary paraganglioma/pheochromocytoma (PGL/PCC). *Neurogenetics.* 2011 Aug;12(3):175-81.

Ozgenc A, Loeb LA. Werner Syndrome, aging and cancer. *Genome Dyn.* 2006;1:206-17

Rosner I, Bratslavsky G, Pinto PA, Linehan WM. The clinical implications of the genetics of renal cell carcinoma. *Urol Oncol.* 2009 Mar-Apr;27(2):131-6.

Rubinstein WS. Endocrine cancer predisposition syndromes: hereditary paraganglioma, multiple endocrine neoplasia type 1, multiple endocrine neoplasia type 2, and hereditary thyroid cancer. *Hematol Oncol Clin North Am.* 2010 Oct;24(5):907-37.

Sabin MA, Werther GA, Kiess W. Genetics of obesity and overgrowth syndromes. *Best Pract Res Clin Endocrinol Metab.* 2011 Feb;25(1):207-20.

Schrader K, Huntsman D. Hereditary diffuse gastric cancer. *Cancer Treat Res.* 2010;155: 33-63.

Segel GB, Lichtman MA. Familial (inherited) leukemia, lymphoma, and myeloma: an overview. *Blood Cells Mol Dis.* 2004 Jan-Feb;32(1):246-61.

Shetty Roy AN, Radin M, Sarabi D, Shaoulian E. Familial recurrent atrial myxoma: Carney's complex. *Clin Cardiol.* 2011 Feb;34(2):83-6.

Su X, Huang J. The Fanconi anemia pathway and DNA interstrand cross-link repair. *Protein Cell.* 2011 Sep;2(9):704-11.

Teplick A, Kowalski M, Biegel JA, Nichols KE. Educational paper: screening in cancer predisposition syndromes: guidelines for the general pediatrician. *Eur J Pediatr.* 2011 Mar;170(3):285-94.

Tomasoni R, Mondino A. The tuberous sclerosis complex: balancing proliferation and survival. *Biochem Soc Trans.* 2011 Apr;39(2):466-71.

Upton B, Chu Q, Li BD. Li-Fraumeni syndrome: the genetics and treatment considerations for the sarcoma and associated neoplasms. *Surg Oncol Clin N Am.* 2009 Jan;18(1):145-56, ix

Weber W, Estoppey J, Stoll H. Familial cancer diagnosis. *Anticancer Res.* 2001 Sep-Oct;21(5):3631-5.

Zbuk KM, Eng C. Hamartomatous polyposis syndromes. *Nat Clin Pract Gastroenterol Hepatol.* 2007 Sep;4(9):492-502.

Chapter 6

Epigenetics and Cancer

Abstract

Epigenetics is defined as heritable changes in gene expression that are not due to any alteration in the DNA sequence. Intense research in the last 20 years has shown that epigenetic regulation of DNA-templated processes (DNA methylation, histone modification, nucleosome remodeling, and RNA-mediated targeting) regulate a number of biological processes that are fundamental to the genesis of cancer.

Introduction

The term "epigenetics" is most commonly used to describe chromatin-based events that regulate DNA-templated processes.

Chromatin is the macromolecular complex of DNA and histone proteins, which provides the scaffold for the packaging of the entire genome. Its basic units are 147 base pairs of DNA wrapped around a histone octamer, with two each of histones H2A, H2B, H3, and H4. Histones and DNA can be chemically modified with epigenetic marks that influence chromatin structure by altering the electrostatic nature of the chromatin and/or by altering the affinity of interactions with chromatin-binding proteins.

Chromatin can be subdivided into two major regions:

- heterochromatin, which is highly condensed, late to replicate, and primarily contains inactive genes;
- euchromatin, which is relatively open and contains most of the active genes.

Euchromatin exhibits lower levels of DNA methylation, relative to heterochromatin, and the nucleosomes in euchromatin contain histones with modifications that promote gene expression.

Epigenetic regulation mainly involves DNA methylation/hydroxymethylation events as well as histone modifications:

Epigenetic Pathways Connected to Cancer

- DNA Methylation
- DNA Hydroxy-Methylation and Its Oxidation Derivatives
- Histone Modifications
    - Histone Acetylation.
    - Histone Deacetylation
    - Histone Acetylation Readers
    - Histone Methylation
    - Histone Demethylation
    - Histone Methylation Readers
    - Histone Phosphorylation

It is now evident that genes encoding proteins involved in these pathways are themselves targeted during tumor initiation and progression.

Epigenetic Pathways Altered in Cancer

DNA Methylation

DNA methylation targets cytosine residues in CpG dinucleotides and is the most extensively characterized modification of chromatin. Global DNA hypomethylation is commonly observed in malignant cells. However, methylation changes that occur within CpG islands, which are present in about 70% of all mammalian promoters, have been more particularly studied. Recent genome-wide maps of CpG methylation have shown that between 5%–10% of normally unmethylated CpG promoter islands become abnormally methylated in various cancer genomes. Moreover, CpG hypermethylation of promoters not only affects the expression of protein coding genes but also the expression of various noncoding RNAs, some of which have a role in malignant transformation (Baylin and Jones, 2011). Of note, while it was previously thought that gene methylation was associated with gene silencing, these studies have established that many actively transcribed genes have high levels of DNA methylation within the gene body, suggesting that the context and spatial distribution of DNA methylation is vital in transcriptional regulation (Baylin and Jones, 2011).

Of the three proteins that were shown to possess catalytic methyltransferase activity (Dnmt1, Dnmt3a, and Dnmt3b). Dnmt1 exhibits a strong preference for hemi-methylated over unmethylated DNA, and its particular targeting of replication foci is thought to allow copying of the parental DNA methylation pattern onto the newly synthesized DNA daughter strand. Therefore, Dnmt1 is regarded as a maintenance methyltransferase. The Dnmt3 family consists of two catalytic members, Dnmt3a and Dnmt3b, both of which exhibit increased methyltransferase activity towards unmethylated over hemi-methylated DNA, which is why they were termed *de novo* methyltransferases. DNMT1 mutations have been found in colorectal cancers (Kanai et al. 2003). DNMT3A mutations are common in *de novo* AML and MDS and are associated with poor survival (Walter et al. 2011)].

DNA Hydroxy-Methylation and Its Oxidation Derivatives

While DNA methylation was long considered to be a relatively stable chromatin modification, the presence of 5-hydroxymethylcytosine (5hmC) in DNA was reported a few years ago (Tahiliani et al. 2009). DNA hydroxylases responsible for catalytically converting 5mC to 5hmC have been identified: the "ten-eleven translocation" (TET) family of proteins, including Tet1, Tet2 and Tet.3. Indeed, iterative oxidation of 5hmC by the TET family results in further oxidation derivatives, including 5-formylcytosine (5fC) and 5-carboxylcytosine (5caC). The biological significance of the 5mC oxidation derivatives is still unclear, but the TET proteins have also been shown to have activating and repressive functions (Wu and Zhang, 2011).

The name "ten-eleven translocation" results from the initial description of a recurrent chromosomal translocation, t(10;11)(q22;q23), which juxtaposes the MLL gene (on chromosome "ten") with TET1 (on chromosome "eleven") in a subset of patients with AML (see chapter "chromosomal alterations"). Recurrent mutations in TET2 have been observed in numerous hematological malignancies (AML, MPD, MDS, CMML). TET2, along with RUNX1, ASXL1 and RAS, is frequently mutated in CMML patients. The clinical implications of TET2 mutations have largely been inconclusive; however, in some subsets of AML patients, TET2 mutations appear to confer a poor prognosis (Patel et al. 2012). Early insights into the process of TET2-mediated oncogenesis have revealed that the patient-associated mutations are largely loss-of-function mutations that consequently result in decreased 5hmC levels and a reciprocal increase in 5mC levels within the malignant cells that harbor them. TET3 is rarely altered in cancer.

Histone Modifications

Histones are subject to diverse posttranslational modifications including phosphorylation, acetylation, methylation, ubiquitination, SUMOylation, ADP ribosylation, deimination, and proline isomerisation. These diverse modifications can modulate the activity of transcription factors, nucleosome remodelers, histone chaperones, and other histone modifiers by altering the chromatin state for either activation or repression. Most of these modifications are dynamic, and the corresponding enzymes include kinases/phosphatases, acetyltransferases /deacetylases, methyltransferases/demethylases, ubiquitin ligases/deubiquitinating enzymes, and SUMO ligases/deSUMOylating enzymes (Miremadi et al. 2007).

This chapter will discuss acetylation, methylation, and phosphorylation, as these modifications have been the most intensively investigated to date.

Histone Acetylation

Acetylation of lysine residues at position N8 is a major histone modification involved in transcription, chromatin structure, and DNA repair. Acetylation neutralizes lysine's positive charge and may consequently weaken the electrostatic interaction between histones and negatively charged DNA. For this reason, histone acetylation is often associated with a more ''open'' chromatin conformation. Consistent with this, histone acetylation is frequently seen at gene promoters and enhancers. Lysine acetylation also serves as the nidus for the binding of various proteins with bromodomain ("BRD") and tandem plant homeodomain ("PHD") fingers, which recognize this modification (Taverna et al. 2007).

Acetylation is highly dynamic and is regulated by the competing activities of two enzymatic families:

- the histone lysine acetyltransferases (HATs or KATs)
- the histone deacetylases (HDACs)

The HATs can be grouped into three main families based on their sequence similarities: Gcn5/PCAF, p300/CBP and the MYST family.

Gen5 and PCAF (p300/CBP-associated factor) can interact with anther HAT-protein complex, i.e., CBP/p300. Both Gcn5/PCAF and p300/CBP acetylate H3 and H4. The HAT activities of CBP/p300 enables the transactivation of DNA binding transcription factors (p53, E2F, myb, GATA1, Rb) as well as the acetylation of all four histone proteins (H2A, H2B, H3, H4). Mutations in the HAT active site inhibit their transcriptional activating function. MYST family proteins acetylate histones H2A, H3, and H4.

HATs were the first enzymes shown to modify histones. It is now clear that many, if not most, of these enzymes have been implicated in neoplastic transformation, and a number of viral oncoproteins are known to associate with them. Mutations in a number of HATs have been observed in solid tumors (colorectal, breast, pancreatic). They may involve the following HATs: p300 (gene EP300), CBP (gene CREBBP), MYST3 (gene MOZ or KAT6A), MYST4 (gene MORF or KAT6B), NCOA1, TIF2 (or NCOA2). Biallelic EP300 mutations have been identified in epithelial tumors. Furthermore, both EP300 and CREBBP, as well as MOZ and MORF, are commonly involved in chromosomal translocations in hematological malignancies, and less commonly in solid tumors (MORF, NCOA1) (MOZ-EP300, MLL-EP300, MLL-CBP, MOZ-CBP, MORF-CBP, MOZ-TIF2, MOZ-NCOA1, PAX3-NCOA1). For instance, MOZ-TIF2 is sufficient to recapitulate an aggressive leukemia in murine models and it can confer stem cell properties and reactivate a self-renewal program when introduced into committed hematopoietic progenitors. It appears that these translocations are involved in leukemogenesis through aberrant acetylation caused by mistargeting of HATs.

Furthermore, altered expression levels of several of the HATs have also been noted in a range of cancers. For instance, NCOA3 is frequently amplified and overexpressed in human breast cancer and behaves as a classical oncogene.

Despite these insights, the great conundrum with regards to unraveling the molecular mechanisms by which histone acetyltransferases contribute to malignant transformation has been dissecting the contribution of altered patterns in acetylation on histone and nonhistone proteins. Although it is clear that global histone acetylation patterns are perturbed in cancers, it is also well established that several nonhistone proteins, including many important oncogenes and tumor suppressors such as MYC, p53, and PTEN, are also dynamically acetylated. A pragmatic view on this issue is that both histone and nonhistone acetylation are likely to be important.

Histone Desacetylation

Histone deacetylases (HDACs) may revert lysine acetylation and restore its positive charge. This consequently strengthens the electrostatic interaction between histones and negatively charged DNA. There are 18 such enzymes identified, and these are subdivided into four major classes, depending on sequence homology:

- Class I (HDAC 1-3 and HDAC8)
- Class II (HDAC 4-7 and HDAC 9-10)
- Class IV (HDAC11).

Class I, II, and IV HDACs share a related catalytic mechanism that requires a zinc metal ion but does not involve the use of a cofactor. In contrast, class III HDACs (sirtuin 1–7) employ a distinct catalytic mechanism that is NAD+-dependent. Analogous to the lysine acetyltransferases, HDACs target both histone and nonhistone proteins. Substrate specificity for these enzymes is largely mediated by components of multisubunit complexes in which HDACs are found, such as Mi2/NuRD, Sin3A, and Co-REST.

Chimeric fusion proteins that are seen in leukemia, such as PML-RARa, PLZF-RARa, and AML1-ETO, have been shown to recruit HDACs to mediate aberrant gene silencing, which contributes to leukemogenesis (Johnstone and Licht, 2003). HDACs can also interact with nonchimeric oncogenes such as BCL6, whose repressive activity is controlled by dynamic acetylation (Bereshchenko et al. 2002).

Most of the HDAC inhibitors (HDAC-I) developed so far are non-selective. Importantly, some of these HDAC inhibitors were shown to change the chromatin structure and cause re-expression of aberrantly silenced genes, which in turn is associated with growth inhibition, differentiation and apoptosis in cancer cells. Based on impressive preclinical and clinical data, two pan-HDAC inhibitors, vorinostat and romidepsin, have been granted FDA approval for clinical use in patients with cutaneous T cell lymphoma. In addition, increasing evidence suggests that combination treatment with inhibitors of HDAC and DNA methyltransferase (DNMT) results in synergy at clinically tolerable doses that may translate not only into changes in methylation but also to disease response.

Germline or somatic mutations in HDACs do not appear to be prominent in cancer. However, the expression levels of various HDACs appear to be altered in numerous malignancies. Consequently, several HDAC–I (entinostat, panobinostat...) are currently under investigation for clinical use in a broad range of cancers. However, the pleiotropic effects of HDACs continue to pose significant challenges in dissecting the specific effects on histone and nonhistone proteins.

Histone Acetylation Readers

The primary readers of N^8-acetylation of lysine residues are families of proteins that contain an evolutionarily conserved binding motif termed a "bromodomain" (BRD). There are over 40 described human proteins with bromodomains. These comprise a diverse group of proteins that function as chromatin remodelers, histone acetyltransferases, histone methyltransferases, and transcriptional coactivators. Many of these proteins also contain several separate evolutionarily conserved "chromatin-reading" motifs such as PHD fingers, which recognize distinct histone posttranslational modifications (Chung and Witherington 2011).

Among histone acetylation readers, some are subject to gene translocation or mutation. For instance, BRD3 and BRD4 may be fused to NUT in midline carcinoma, a rare, very aggressive, poorly-differentiated and invariably fatal cancer. Both BRD3-NUT and BRD4-NUT fusion proteins contain almost the entirety of NUT and are strictly nuclear (French CA, 2010). The gene encoding another acetylation reader, TRIM33 is fused to RET (a protein kinase) in some childhood papillary thyroid carcinomas (Klugbauer and Rabes 1999). PBRM1, encoding Polybromo-1 protein is mutated in breast cancer (Thompson 2009).

The conserved BRD fold contains a deep, largely hydrophobic acetyl lysine binding site, which represents an attractive pocket for the development of small, pharmaceutically active molecules. Recently, potent and selective inhibitors that target BRDs of the BET (bromodomains and extra-terminal) family provided compelling data supporting targeting of these BRDs in inflammation and in cancer (Muller et al. 2011). The BET inhibitors have recently been shown to be efficient in squamous cell carcinoma, in NUT-midline carcinoma and in a range of hematological malignancies. BET proteins play a fundamental role in transcriptional elongation and cell-cycle progression.

Histone Methylation

Histones are methylated on the side chains of arginine, lysine, and histidine residues. Methylation, unlike acetylation and phosphorylation, does not alter the overall charge of the molecule. Lysines may be mono-, di-, or tri-methylated, and arginine residues may be symmetrically or asymmetrically methylated. The best-characterized sites of histone methylation are those that occur on lysine residues and, therefore, these will be the focus of this section. Although many lysine residues on the various histones are methylated, the best studied are H3K4, H3K9, H3K27, H3K36, H3K79, and H4K20. Some of these (H3K4, H3K36, and H3K79) are often associated with active genes in euchromatin, whereas others (H3K9, H3K27, and H4K20) are associated with heterochromatic regions of the genome. Different methylation states on the same residue can also localize differently. For instance, H3K4me2/3 usually spans the transcriptional start site (TSS) of active genes, whereas H3K4me1 is a modification associated with active enhancers. Similarly, whereas monomethylation of H3K9 may be seen at active genes, trimethylation of H3K9 is associated with gene repression (Barski et al. 2007).

The enzymatic protagonists for lysine methylation contain a conserved SET domain, which possesses methyltransferase activity. In contrast to the KATs, the histone lysine methyltransferases (KMT) tend to be highly specific enzymes that specifically target certain lysine residues. Recurrent translocations and/or coding mutations have been found in a large number of KMT.

MLL (also KMT2A), located on 11q23, which is recurrent locus of chromosomal translocation in AML and ALL, has been found in more than 50 translocations with fusion partners, and cases with MLL translocations are generally associated with an intermediate to poor prognosis (Krivtsov and Armstrong 2007). Partial tandem duplications (PTDs) of MLL have also been observed in acute leukemias with trisomy of chromosome 11 or normal karyotype. MLL2 (also KMT2B) is altered in medulloblastoma, prostate cancer, DLBCL, FL. MLL3 (also KMT2C) is altered in breast, liver, gastric, colorectal and in hematological malignancies. SETD2 (KMT3A) is frequently mutated in clear cell renal cancer.

Regarding EZH2 (also KMT6), both its overexpression and its inactivation have been associated to cancer. Whether EZH2 is an oncogene or a tumor suppressor remains unclear. Heterozygous missense mutations resulting in the substitution of tyrosine 641 (Y641) within the SET domain of EZH2 were noted in DLBCL (Morin et al. 2010). This mutation was shown to increase EZH2 catalytic activity and a preference for converting H3K27me1 to H3K27me2/3, supporting the contention that EZH2 is an oncogene (Sneeringer et al. 2010). In contrast, loss-of-function mutations in EZH2 gene, conferring a poor prognosis, have been described in the myeloid malignancies (Ernst et al. 2010; Nikoloski et al. 2010) and T-ALL (Ntziachristos et al. 2012; Zhang et al. 2012), suggesting a tumor-suppressive role for EZH2 in these cell lineages.

Among the members of the RIZ family of HMTs, PRDM1 (also known as BLIMP1) is mutated in DLBCL, PRDM3 (also known as MECOM) and PRDM16 are involved in translocations.

Among the members of SET2 family, NSD1 (nuclear receptor binding SET domain protein 1) (also known as KMT3B) is involved in translocations with a nucleoporin gene (NUP98) to produce a fusion protein in childhood AML, NSD2 is the gene disrupted by the t(4:14) in MM producing an IgH/NSD2 hybrid transcript resulting in overexpression of transcripts originating from the NSD2. NSD3 is amplified in human breast cancer cell lines and primary tumors, and subsequently was identified at the breakpoint of t(8;11)(p11.2;p15), resulting in a fusion of the NUP98 and NSD genes.

Histone Demethylation

Two classes of histone demethylases have been identified. The first class includes LSD1 (lysine-specific demethylase 1) which can reverse histone H3K4 and H3K9 modifications by an oxidative demethylation reaction. As this family of enzymes requires protonated nitrogen to initiate demethylation, they are limited to demethylating mono- and dimethyllysine. The second and more expansive class of enzymes is broadly referred to as the Jumonji demethylases.

Thus far, recurrent coding mutations have been noted in KDM5A (JARID1A), KDM5C (JARID1C), and KDM6A (UTX). Mutations in UTX, in particular, are prevalent in a large number of solid and hematological cancers. Small-molecule inhibitors of the two families of histone demethylases are at various stages of development, and this interest will be spurred on by emerging preclinical data showing the therapeutic potential of compounds that inhibit LSD1/KDM1A in AML (Barretina et al. 2012; Schenk et al. 2012).

While the expression of various HMT may be modified in cancer, genetic alterations have been observed only for KDM4C (JMJD2C), KDM5A (JARID1A), KDM5C (JARID1C) and KDM6A (UTX). KDM4C is amplified in prostate cancer, esophageal squamous cell carcinoma, desmoplastic medulloblastoma, metastatic lung sarcomatoid carcinoma, mucosa-associated lymphoid tissue (MALT) lymphoma, and breast cancer; KDM5A is involved in translocations leading to a NUP98-JARID1A fusion protein in AML; KDM5C is mutated in renal cancer. Mutations in KDM6A (UTX) are prevalent in a large number of solid and hematological cancers.

Small-molecule inhibitors of the two families of histone demethylases are at various stages of development.

Histone Methylation Readers

The various states of lysine methylation result in considerable physicochemical diversity of lysine; these modification states are read and interpreted by proteins containing different specialized recognition motifs. Broadly speaking, the aromatic cages that engage methyllysine can be divided into two major families, the Royal Family (Tudor domains, Chromo domains, and malignant brain tumor [MBT] domains) and PHD fingers (Taverna et al. 2007).

Several methyllysine readers have also been implicated in cancer, although their role in the disease remains elusive. For instance, ING family members have coding mutations identified in malignancies such as melanoma, breast cancer, and HNSCC, including those that specifically target the PHD finger, which recognizes H3K4me3 (Coles and Jones 2009).

Histone Phosphorylation

Histone may be phosphorylated at serine, threonine, and tyrosine residues; This alters the charge of the protein, which influences overall structure and function of the local chromatin environment. Phosphorylation is a highly dynamic process, which is reciprocally controlled by the competing activities of protein kinases and protein phosphatases (removing phosphate residues).

At the global cellular level, kinases are the main orchestrators of signal transduction pathways conveying extracellular cues within the cell. Alterations involving signaling kinases are some of the most frequent oncogenic phenomena described in cancer (Hanahan and Weinberg 2011).

While many kinases have established roles as signal transducers in the cytoplasm; however, it has recently been recognized that some kinases may also have nuclear functions, which include the phosphorylation of histones (for a review, see (Baek et al. 2011)). Some of these histone kinases also act on transcription factors and histone modifiers.

An interesting example of histone-phosphorylating kinase is the nonreceptor tyrosine kinase, JAK2, since it is frequently amplified or mutated in the hematological malignancies (myeloproliferative neoplasms, leukemia). JAK2 is well-known to phosphorylate signal transducer and activator of transcription 5 (STAT5). In addition, within the nucleus, JAK2 specifically phosphorylates H3Y41, disrupts the binding of the chromatin repressor heterochromatin protein 1α (HP1α), and triggers increased expression of oncogenic transcription factors, such as LMO2, enhanced mitotic recombination, chromosomal disjunction and aneuploidy (Dawson et al., 2009). It has been shown recently that the JAK2 and JMJD2C genes, both located at 9p24, could be co-amplified in primary mediastinal B-cell lymphoma (PMBL) and Hodgkin lymphoma (HL). JMJD2C encodes a histone demethylase and it appears that both JAK2 and JMJD2C cooperatively remodel the PMBL and HL epigenome (Rui et al. 2010).

Given that many small-molecule inhibitors against kinases are clinically used as anticancer therapies, it is interesting to note that several of these (e.g., JAK2 and Aurora inhibitors) result in a global reduction in the histone modifications laid down by these enzymes. These agents can therefore be considered as potential epigenetic therapies.

Protein phosphatases, like protein kinases, demonstrate specificity for either serine/threonine residues or tyrosine residues, or they may have dual specificity. Little is currently known about the function of these enzymes at chromatin and their potential misadventures in cancer.

Cancer Mutations in Histone Genes

Recent studies have identified somatic mutations in the histone H3.3-coding gene (H3F3A) and in the canonical histone H3.1 (HIST1H3B) in a large proportion of pediatric glioblastomas (Khuong-Quang et al. 2012). They were the first somatic mutations described in histone genes. These mutations are invariably heterozygous and are clustered such that they primarily result in amino acid substitutions at two critical residues in the tail of histone H3 (K27M, G34R/G34V). By virtue of the residues they disrupt, these mutations are likely to have an important influence on chromatin structure and transcription. For instance, the K27M mutation alters the ability of this critical residue to be both methylated and acetylated. These posttranslational modifications of H3K27 have different genomic distributions within euchromatin and heterochromatin; they are recognized by different epigenetic readers and are ultimately associated with different transcriptional outcomes.

Chromatin Remodelers

The myriad of covalent modifications on the nucleosome often provides the scaffold and context for dynamic ATP-dependent chromatin remodeling. Based on their biochemical activity and subunit composition, the mammalian chromatin-remodeling complexes can be broadly split into four major families (Brien and Bracken 2009):

- the switching defective/sucrose nonfermenting (SWI/SNF) family
- the imitation SWI (ISWI) family
- the nucleosome remodeling and deacetylation (NuRD)/Mi-2/chromodomain helicase DNA binding (CHD) family
- the inositol requiring 80 (INO80) family.

These enzymes are involved in mobilization, eviction, and exchange of histones. Each of these families is characterized by specific domain structures and is populated by members that contain various chromatin reader motifs (SANT domains, bromodomains, and chromodomains) that confer some regional and context specificity to their chromatin-remodeling activities (Wang et al. 2007).

Various members of chromatin-remodeling families have been associated to cancer. This is notably the case for MTA1 (metastasis associated gene 1), which encodes a critical component of the nucleosome remodeling and histone deacetylase (NuRD) complex, express a dual corepressor or coactivator nature and is widely overexpressed in human cancers (Li et al. 2012). MTA1 expression correlates with tumor formation in the mammary gland. In addition, MTA1 converts breast cancer cells to a more aggressive phenotype by repression of the estrogen receptor (ER) α trans-activation function through deacetylation of the chromatin in the ER-responsive element of ER-α-responsive genes. Furthermore, MTA1 plays an essential role in c-MYC-mediated cell transformation.

To date, most mutations affecting members of chromatin-remodeling families have been described in components of the SWI/SNF complex, which plays essential roles in a variety of cellular processes including differentiation, proliferation and DNA repair. It is suggested to function as a tumor suppressor. Genes encoding components of the SWI/SNF complex include ARID1A (AT rich interactive domain 1A (SWI-like)), ARID1B, ARID2, SMARCA2 (SWI/SNF related, matrix associated, actin dependent regulator of chromatin, subfamily a, member 2), SMARCA4, SMARCB1, SMARCC1, SMARCC2, SMARCD1, SMARCD2, SMARCD3, SMARCE1, ACTL6A (Actin-like 6A), ACTL6B, and PBRM1 (Polybromo 1)

Among these genes, ARID1A (1p36.1-p35), ARID1B (6q25.3), ARID2 (12q13.11), PBRM1 (3p21), SMARCA4 (19p13.3) and SMARCB1 (22q11.23) are the most frequently mutated components of the SWI/SNF complex in a range of hematological and solid malignancies. The prevalence of these mutations would suggest that many of the members of these complexes are involved in the development and maintenance of cancer; however, functional insights into the mechanisms of oncogenesis are only just beginning to emerge. It is clear that the SWI/SNF complexes have several lineage-specific subunits and interact with tissue-specific transcription factors to regulate differentiation. They also have a reciprocal and antagonistic relationship with the polycomb complexes. One possibility, which remains to be formally established, is that mutations in SWI/SNF members potentiate malignancy by skewing the balance between self-renewal and differentiation.

Genetic evidence from mouse models has confirmed that altered expression of these purported tumor suppressors can increase the propensity to develop cancer. In the case of SMARCA4, even haploinsufficiency results in increased tumors (Wilson and Roberts 2011).

Noncoding RNAs

The high-throughput genomic platforms have established that virtually the entire genome is transcribed; however, only ~2% of this is subsequently translated (Amaral et al. 2008). The remaining "noncoding" RNAs (ncRNAs) can be roughly categorized into small (under 200 nucleotides) and long ncRNAs. Long ncRNAs (lncRNAs) appear to have a critical function at chromatin, where they may act as molecular chaperones or scaffolds for various chromatin regulators, and their function may be subverted in cancer (Wang and Chang 2011).

One of the best-studied lncRNAs is HOTAIR (HOX Antisense Intergenic RNA), a 2.2 kb lncRNA transcribed in antisense direction from the HOXC gene cluster. HOTAIR functions in trans by interacting and recruiting the chromatin-modifying "polycomb repressive complex 2" (PRC2) to the HOXD locus which leads to transcriptional silencing across 40 kb. HOTAIR also interact with a second histone modification complex, the LSD1/CoREST/REST complex, which coordinates targeting of PRC2 and LSD1 to chromatin for coupled histone H3K27 methylation and K4 demethylation.

Given its important role in the epigenetic regulation of gene expression, it is not surprising that HOTAIR is deregulated in different types of cancer (breast, liver). In human breast cancer, HOTAIR expression is increased in primary tumors and metastases and its expression level in primary tumors positively correlates with metastasis and poor outcome. Overexpression of HOTAIR in epithelial cancer cells alters H3K27 methylation via PRC2 and therefore alters target gene expression. This leads to increased cancer invasiveness and metastases. On the other hand, HOTAIR depletion inhibits cancer invasiveness. Similar to breast cancer, HOTAIR depletion in liver cancer cells reduces cell invasion and cell viability. Moreover, HOTAIR might be a potential biomarker for the existence of lymph node metastasis in HCC. In addition, HOTAIR suppression sensitizes cancer cells to tumor necrosis factor-α induced apoptosis and renders them more sensitive to the chemotherapeutic agents cisplatin and doxorubicin.

Conclusion

The principal tenet in oncology—that cancer is a disease initiated and driven by genetic anomalies—remains uncontested, but it is now clear that deregulation of epigenetic pathways also play a significant role in oncogenesis. Further understanding of the epigenetic regulation of tissue-specific genes along with the development of more specific epigenetic drugs may hold the key to our ability to successfully reset the abnormal cancer epigenome.

References

Baek SH. When signaling kinases meet histones and histone modifiers in the nucleus. *Mol Cell.* 2011 May 6;42(3):274-84.

Barretina J, Caponigro G, Stransky N, Venkatesan K, Margolin AA, Kim S, Wilson CJ, Lehár J, Kryukov GV, Sonkin D, et al. The Cancer Cell Line Encyclopedia enables predictive modelling of anticancer drug sensitivity. Nature. 2012 Mar 28;483(7391):603-7.

Barski A, Cuddapah S, Cui K, Roh TY, Schones DE, Wang Z, Wei G, Chepelev I, Zhao K. High-resolution profiling of histone methylations in the human genome. *Cell.* 2007 May 18;129(4):823-37.

Baylin SB, Jones PA. A decade of exploring the cancer epigenome - biological and translational implications. *Nat Rev Cancer.* 2011 Sep 23;11(10):726-34.

Bereshchenko OR, Gu W, Dalla-Favera R. Acetylation inactivates the transcriptional repressor BCL6. *Nat Genet.* 2002 Dec;32(4):606-13.

Brien GL, Bracken AP. Transcriptomics: unravelling the biology of transcription factors and chromatin remodelers during development and differentiation. *Semin Cell Dev Biol.* 2009 Sep;20(7):835-41.

Chung CW, Witherington J. Progress in the discovery of small-molecule inhibitors of bromodomain--histone interactions. *J Biomol Screen.* 2011 Dec;16(10):1170-85.

Coles AH, Jones SN. The ING gene family in the regulation of cell growth and tumorigenesis. *J Cell Physiol.* 2009 Jan;218(1):45-57.

Dawson MA, Bannister AJ, Göttgens B, Foster SD, Bartke T, Green AR, Kouzarides T. JAK2 phosphorylates histone H3Y41 and excludes HP1alpha from chromatin. *Nature.* 2009 Oct 8;461(7265):819-22.

Ernst T, Chase AJ, Score J, Hidalgo-Curtis CE, Bryant C, Jones AV, Waghorn K, Zoi K, Ross FM, Reiter A, et al. Inactivating mutations of the histone methyltransferase gene EZH2 in myeloid disorders. *Nat Genet.* 2010 Aug;42(8):722-6.

French CA. NUT midline carcinoma. *Cancer Genet Cytogenet.* 2010 Nov;203(1):16-20.

Hanahan D, Weinberg RA. Hallmarks of cancer: the next generation. *Cell.* 2011 Mar 4;144(5):646-74.

Johnstone RW, Licht JD. Histone deacetylase inhibitors in cancer therapy: is transcription the primary target? *Cancer Cell.* 2003 Jul;4(1):13-8.

Kanai Y, Ushijima S, Nakanishi Y, Sakamoto M, Hirohashi S. Mutation of the DNA methyltransferase (DNMT) 1 gene in human colorectal cancers. *Cancer Lett.* 2003 Mar 20;192(1):75-82.

Klugbauer S, Rabes HM. The transcription coactivator HTIF1 and a related protein are fused to the RET receptor tyrosine kinase in childhood papillary thyroid carcinomas. *Oncogene.* 1999 Jul 29;18(30):4388-93.

Khuong-Quang DA, Buczkowicz P, Rakopoulos P, Liu XY, Fontebasso AM, Bouffet E, Bartels U, Albrecht S, Schwartzentruber J, Letourneau L, et al. K27M mutation in histone H3.3 defines clinically and biologically distinct subgroups of pediatric diffuse intrinsic pontine gliomas. *Acta Neuropathol.* 2012 Sep;124(3):439-47.

Krivtsov AV, Armstrong SA. MLL translocations, histone modifications and leukaemia stem-cell development. *Nat Rev Cancer.* 2007 Nov;7(11):823-33.

Li DQ, Pakala SB, Nair SS, Eswaran J, Kumar R. Metastasis-associated protein 1/nucleosome remodeling and histone deacetylase complex in cancer. *Cancer Res.* 2012 Jan 15;72(2):387-94.

Miremadi A, Oestergaard MZ, Pharoah PD, Caldas C. Cancer genetics of epigenetic genes. *Hum Mol Genet.* 2007 Apr 15;16 Spec No 1:R28-49.

Muller S, Filippakopoulos P, Knapp S. Bromodomains as therapeutic targets. *Expert Rev Mol Med.* 2011 Sep 13;13:e29.

Nikoloski G, Langemeijer SM, Kuiper RP, Knops R, Massop M, Tönnissen ER, van der Heijden A, Scheele TN, Vandenberghe P, de Witte T, et al. Somatic mutations of the histone methyltransferase gene EZH2 in myelodysplastic syndromes. *Nat Genet.* 2010 Aug;42(8):665-7.

Ntziachristos P, Tsirigos A, Van Vlierberghe P, Nedjic J, Trimarchi T, Flaherty MS, Ferres-Marco D, da Ros V, Tang Z, Siegle J, et al. Genetic inactivation of the polycomb repressive complex 2 in T cell acute lymphoblastic leukemia. *Nat Med.* 2012 Feb 6;18(2):298-301.

Patel JP, Gönen M, Figueroa ME, Fernandez H, Sun Z, Racevskis J, Van Vlierberghe P, Dolgalev I, Thomas S, Aminova O, et al. Prognostic relevance of integrated genetic profiling in acute myeloid leukemia. *N Engl J Med.* 2012 Mar 22;366(12):1079-89.

Rui L, Emre NC, Kruhlak MJ, Chung HJ, Steidl C, Slack G, Wright GW, Lenz G, Ngo VN, Shaffer AL, et al. Cooperative epigenetic modulation by cancer amplicon genes. *Cancer Cell.* 2010 Dec 14;18(6):590-605.

Schenk T, Chen WC, Göllner S, Howell L, Jin L, Hebestreit K, Klein HU, Popescu AC, Burnett A, Mills K, et al. Inhibition of the LSD1 (KDM1A) demethylase reactivates the all-trans-retinoic acid differentiation pathway in acute myeloid leukemia. *Nat Med.* 2012 Mar 11;18(4):605-11.

Sneeringer CJ, Scott MP, Kuntz KW, Knutson SK, Pollock RM, Richon VM, Copeland RA. Coordinated activities of wild-type plus mutant EZH2 drive tumor-associated hypertrimethylation of lysine 27 on histone H3 (H3K27) in human B-cell lymphomas. *Proc Natl Acad Sci U S A.* 2010 Dec 7;107(49):20980-5.

Tahiliani M, Koh KP, Shen Y, Pastor WA, Bandukwala H, Brudno Y, Agarwal S, Iyer LM, Liu DR, Aravind L, Rao A. Conversion of 5-methylcytosine to 5-hydroxymethylcytosine in mammalian DNA by MLL partner TET1. *Science.* 2009 May 15;324(5929):930-5.

Taverna SD, Li H, Ruthenburg AJ, Allis CD, Patel DJ. How chromatin-binding modules interpret histone modifications: lessons from professional pocket pickers. *Nat Struct Mol Biol.* 2007 Nov;14(11):1025-40.

Thompson M. Polybromo-1: the chromatin targeting subunit of the PBAF complex. *Biochimie.* 2009 Mar;91(3):309-19.

Walter MJ, Ding L, Shen D, Shao J, Grillot M, McLellan M, Fulton R, Schmidt H, Kalicki-Veizer J, O'Laughlin M, et al. Recurrent DNMT3A mutations in patients with myelodysplastic syndromes. *Leukemia.* 2011 Jul;25(7):1153-8.

Wang GG, Allis CD, Chi P. Chromatin remodeling and cancer, Part II: ATP-dependent chromatin remodeling. *Trends Mol Med.* 2007 Sep;13(9):373-80.

Wang KC, Chang HY. Molecular mechanisms of long noncoding RNAs. *Mol Cell.* 2011 Sep 16;43(6):904-14.

Wilson BG, Roberts CW. SWI/SNF nucleosome remodellers and cancer. *Nat Rev Cancer.* 2011 Jun 9;11(7):481-92.

Wu H, Zhang Y. Mechanisms and functions of Tet protein-mediated 5-methylcytosine oxidation. *Genes Dev.* 2011 Dec 1;25(23):2436-52.

Zhang J, Ding L, Holmfeldt L, Wu G, Heatley SL, Payne-Turner D, Easton J, Chen X, Wang J, Rusch M, et al. The genetic basis of early T-cell precursor acute lymphoblastic leukaemia. *Nature.* 2012 Jan 11;481(7380):157-63.

Abbreviations

Abbreviation	Term
AEL	Acute eosinophilic leukemia
AL	Acute leukemia
ALCL	Anaplastic large-cell lymphoma
ALL	Acute lymphocytic leukemia
AML	Acute myelogenous leukemia
AML^t	Acute myelogenous leukemia (primarily treatment associated)
APL	Acute promyelocytic leukemia
B-ALL	B-cell acute lymphocytic leukaemia
B-CLL	B-cell Lymphocytic leukemia
B-NHL	B-cell Non-Hodgkin Lymphoma
BCC	Basal cell carcinoma
BCP-ALL	B-cell precursor acute lymphoblastic leukemia
CEL	Chronic eosinophilic leukemia
CLL	Chronic lymphatic leukemia
CML	Chronic myeloid leukemia
CMML	Chronic myelomonocytic leukemia
CNS	Central nervous system
DFSP	Dermatofibrosarcoma protuberans
DLBCL	Diffuse large B-cell lymphoma
DLCL	Diffuse large-cell lymphoma
EMS	8p11 myeloproliferative syndrome
FL	Follicular lymphoma
GIST	Gastrointestinal stromal tumour
HL	Hodgkin lymphoma
HNPCC	Hereditary non-polyposis colorectal cancer
IMT	Inflammatory myofibroblastic tumor
JMML	Juvenile myelomonocytic leukemia
MALT	Mucosa-associated lymphoid tissue lymphoma
MDS	Myelodysplastic syndrome
MDS^t	Myelodysplastic syndrome (primarily treatment associated)
MLCLS	Mediastinal large cell lymphoma with sclerosis
MM	Multiple myeloma

MPD	Myeloproliferative disorder
MPS	Myeloproliferative syndrome
NHL	Non-Hodgkin lymphoma
NK/T	Natural killer T cell
NSCLC	Non small cell lung cancer
PMBL	Primary mediastinal B-cell lymphoma
PNET	Primitive neurectodermal tumors
pre-B All	Pre-B-cell acute lymphoblastic leukaemia
PTCL	Peripheral T-cell lymphoma
RAEB	Refractory anemia with excess blasts
RAEB[t]	Refractory anemia with excess blasts (primarily treatment associated)
RCC	Renal cell carcinoma
SCC	Squamous cell carcinoma
SLL	Small lymphocytic lymphoma
T-ALL	T-cell acute lymphoblastic leukemia
T-CLL	T-cell chronic lymphocytic leukaemia
TGCT	Testicular germ cell tumour
T-PLL	T cell prolymphocytic leukaemia

Index

#

10q23, 8, 49, 50, 123, 126, 141
10q24, 59
9p24, 30, 127, 174

A

ABL1, 2, 70, 73, 75, 76, 82, 83, 89, 90, 95
access, 38
accounting, 116, 137, 148
acetylation, x, 38, 169, 170, 171, 172
acid, 3, 5, 19, 21, 36, 179
acidic, 23, 124
acoustic neuroma, 39, 155
ACTH, 47, 152
active site, 170
acute leukemia, 62, 69, 80, 139, 146, 172
acute lymphoblastic leukemia, 2, 16, 25, 64, 72, 94, 95, 128, 178, 181, 182
acute myeloblastic leukemia, 159
acute myelogenous leukemia, 142, 143
acute myeloid leukemia, 2, 12, 22, 25, 40, 54, 96, 104, 143, 144, 178, 179
acute promyelocytic leukemia, 41
AD, 69, 71, 112, 165
adenine, 37, 128
adenocarcinoma, 9, 49, 50, 59, 64, 79, 82, 86, 93, 94, 101, 131, 143, 146, 148
adenoma, 5, 66, 79, 81, 82, 84, 85, 86, 150, 157
adenomatous polyposis coli, 17
adenosine, 58
adhesion(s), 2, 4, 13, 14, 17, 19
adhesive interaction, 13
adipocyte, 16, 105
ADP, 169
adrenal gland, 5, 17, 19, 28, 33, 53, 151
adrenal glands, 17, 19, 33, 151
adulthood, 7, 18, 24, 39, 69
adults, 38
aerodigestive tract, 5, 6, 12, 15, 29, 38, 40, 57, 123, 128, 142
aflatoxin, 64
age, 4, 7, 9, 10, 35, 39, 49, 51, 63, 64, 67, 68, 135, 137, 138, 139, 142, 143, 144, 146, 147, 148, 150, 151, 152, 154, 155, 156, 157, 160, 161, 163, 164
aggregation, 115
aggressiveness, 102, 108, 110
AKT1, 2, 3
AKT2, 2, 3, 98, 100, 112
alanine, 142
aldehydes, 21
aldosterone, 152
ALK, 3, 4, 41, 76, 79, 82, 83, 84, 93
allele, 14, 24, 48, 50, 58, 64, 116, 124, 129, 133
ALT, 173
alters, 174, 175, 177
amino acid(s), 2, 3, 4, 5, 7, 8, 13, 17, 19, 20, 22, 23, 24, 25, 26, 27, 28, 29, 31, 32, 36, 39, 40, 41, 43, 44, 46, 49, 50, 53, 56, 59, 66, 69, 122, 142, 175
ampulla, 143
anchorage, 44, 108
androgen, 77
anemia, 9, 10, 11, 21, 25, 54, 62, 71, 73, 95, 144, 166, 182
aneuploid, 12
aneuploidy, 11, 97, 108, 165, 174
angiogenesis, 2, 3, 31, 100, 120, 149, 161
angioimmunoblastic T-cell lymphoma, 92
aniridia, 69
anorexia, 163
anther, 170
antibody, 96
anticancer drug, 177
antigen, 9, 77, 120, 124, 132

antisense, 128, 176
APC, 4, 5, 17, 22, 37, 72, 115, 120, 142, 143, 153
APL, 91, 93, 94, 181
aplastic anemia, 159
apoptosis, 4, 5, 6, 12, 16, 17, 31, 34, 37, 58, 62, 63, 65, 102, 105, 106, 113, 122, 128, 133, 141, 151, 152, 161, 171, 177
AR, 98, 101, 165, 178
arginine, 14, 172
ARPC1A, 98, 101, 111
arrest, 5, 15, 17, 34, 51, 58, 63, 106, 119, 123, 136, 141, 150
Ashkenazi Jews, 139
aspartic acid, 12, 18
astrocytoma(s), 9, 15, 31, 154, 155
ASXL1, 46, 62, 81, 169
ataxia, 6, 7, 135, 137
Ataxia Telangiectasia, 5, 136
atherosclerosis, 68, 69
ATM, 5, 6, 7, 34, 70, 115, 116, 136, 137, 145, 155
ATP, 7, 24, 66, 67, 175, 179
atrial myxoma, 166
atrophy, 24, 52
AURKA, 98, 107
autopsy, 161, 162
autosomal dominant, 5, 7, 8, 15, 18, 20, 24, 33, 34, 36, 39, 45, 48, 49, 50, 51, 52, 55, 57, 58, 63, 65, 69, 121, 135, 136, 137, 138, 139, 140, 141, 142, 143, 144, 146, 147, 148, 149, 150, 152, 153, 154, 156, 157, 158, 160, 161, 163
autosomal recessive, 7, 10, 11, 37, 48, 52, 68, 136, 139, 141, 144, 153, 158, 159, 161, 162, 164
avoidance, 72
axial skeleton, 147

B

BAP1, 6, 61, 70, 72
basal cell carcinoma, 18, 48, 49, 64, 70, 128, 137, 159, 165
Basal Cell Nevus Syndrome, 48, 137
base, 24, 26, 34, 37, 51, 153, 167
base pair, 24, 167
BCL2L2, 98, 101
BD, 166
Beckwith–Wiedemann Syndrome, 138
Belgium, x
benign, 15, 17, 18, 20, 23, 24, 28, 35, 39, 44, 45, 48, 49, 55, 58, 61, 64, 65, 106, 120, 137, 138, 139, 140, 141, 142, 143, 144, 145, 146, 147, 148, 149, 150, 151, 152, 153, 154, 155, 156, 157, 158, 159, 160, 161, 162, 163, 164
benign tumors, 39, 49, 55, 61, 64, 139, 162

bicarbonate, 118
Bilateral, 135
bile, 10, 25, 28, 40, 41, 149
bile duct, 10, 25, 40, 41, 149
biliary tract, 14, 15, 23, 32, 57, 128, 148
biological processes, 167
biosynthesis, 20
Birt–Hogg–Dubé Syndrome, 138
births, 39, 50, 51, 53, 58, 136, 137, 138, 139, 141, 144, 147, 152, 156, 157, 159, 160, 162, 163, 164
bladder cancer, 23, 29, 103, 124, 129, 130
bleeding, 39, 50
BLM, 7, 139
blood, 6, 26, 62, 136, 143, 161
blood vessels, 6, 136, 161
Bloom Syndrome, 7, 139
BMPR1A, 7, 8, 50, 121, 156, 157
bone(s), 7, 10, 20, 23, 28, 31, 50, 52, 61, 62, 63, 65, 78, 83, 85, 89, 91, 93, 117, 120, 132, 137, 140, 141, 142, 143, 147, 151, 159
bone cancer, 65
bone marrow, 10, 31, 62, 141, 142, 143, 159
bone tumors, 20, 147
bowel, x, 141, 148, 157
BRAF, 8, 9, 14, 60, 79, 80, 82, 86
brain, 5, 29, 36, 45, 63, 64, 65, 106, 143, 144, 150, 151, 154, 158, 160, 164, 174
brain cancer, 63, 150
brain tumor, 29, 45, 63, 64, 106, 143, 144, 151, 158, 160, 164, 174
BRCA1, 6, 7, 9, 10, 11, 21, 34, 51, 64, 70, 73, 115, 116, 124, 131, 136, 144, 145
BRCA2, 9, 10, 11, 17, 21, 22, 42, 51, 73, 115, 116, 118, 144, 145
breast carcinoma, 14, 42, 76, 92, 99, 111
BRIP1, 11, 21, 22, 70, 116, 144
bromodomains, 171, 172, 175
bronchus, 151
BUB1B, 11, 161

C

Ca^{2+}, 13, 58, 101
CACNA1E, 98, 101, 112
cafe au lait spots, 5
cafe-au-lait spots, 39
calcium, 117, 137
cancer cells, 97, 102, 106, 109, 121, 146, 171, 177
cancer death, 105
cancer progression, 109
candidates, 129
carcinogen, 64, 124, 130
carcinogenesis, 31, 40, 120

carcinoid tumor, 151
Carney Complex, Types I and II, 140
cartilage, 20
cascades, 19, 25, 32
CASP8, 12, 116, 117, 118, 126
Caspase-8, 71
caspases, 12
catalytic activity, 37, 173
cataract, 52
cation, 130
Caucasians, 37, 105
causation, 96
CBFB, 12, 73, 80, 81, 82, 93
CBL, 13, 72, 81, 90
CBP, 170
CCND1, 3, 14, 80, 84, 90, 91, 98, 101, 120, 121
CCND2, 14, 84, 88, 91, 92
CCNE1, 98, 102, 124, 125
CDH1, 13, 14, 72, 120, 121, 145, 146
CDK inhibitor, 15
CDK4, 14, 15, 98, 102, 109, 112, 113
CDKN2A, 1, 14, 15, 16, 40, 63, 89, 117, 125, 126, 128
CEBPA, 16, 92
cell biology, 27
cell cycle, 2, 5, 10, 14, 15, 16, 33, 34, 37, 49, 51, 58, 63, 76, 101, 102, 103, 104, 105, 106, 108, 109, 119, 123, 128, 136, 141, 157, 161
cell death, 107, 123
cell differentiation, 2
cell division, ix, 8, 51, 74, 158
cell fate, 38
cell invasion, 177
cell invasiveness, 13
cell line(s), 3, 23, 52, 59, 61, 62, 63, 78, 85, 96, 100, 101, 105, 106, 107, 108, 112, 124, 128, 133, 173
cell metabolism, 2, 65, 70
cell signaling, 117
cell surface, 19, 42, 124
cellular energy, 146
central nervous system (CNS), 1, 15, 19, 20, 27, 39, 40, 43, 46, 49, 54, 61, 94, 107, 112, 128, 137, 158, 161, 181
centriole, 160
centrosome, 40, 108
cerebellum, 49, 59
cervical cancer, 23, 64, 144
cervix, 10, 23, 29, 44, 58, 139, 156
challenges, 72, 171
chaperones, 169, 176
CHD1L, 98, 102, 110
CHEK2, 10, 16, 17, 63, 89, 115, 116, 136, 145, 150
chemical(s), 124, 125, 130

chemotherapeutic agent, 177
chemotherapy, 102, 107, 108, 111, 113, 145
childhood, 7, 11, 22, 39, 41, 43, 51, 61, 63, 139, 143, 158, 159, 160, 163, 172, 173, 178
childhood cancer, 63
children, 26, 39, 59, 69, 136, 137, 138, 143, 154, 163
chondroma, 85
chondrosarcoma, 20, 78, 85, 89, 147, 150
choroid, 64, 158
chromosomal abnormalities, 77
chromosomal alterations, 103, 169
chromosomal instability, 7, 142, 143, 146, 159
chromosome, 8, 11, 20, 45, 48, 50, 52, 75, 77, 79, 82, 96, 98, 108, 113, 131, 137, 138, 150, 155, 158, 169, 172
chromosome 10, 8, 50, 96
chromosome 11p11.2, 20
chronic lymphocytic leukemia, 6, 129, 137
chronic obstructive pulmonary disease, 122
cilia, 122, 130
CKS1B, 98, 102
classes, 45, 171, 173
cleavage, 34
cleft lip, 127
clinical diagnosis, 138, 142
clinical presentation, 165
clinical symptoms, 62
clustering, 38, 118
clusters, 45
CO2, 24
coding, 1, 3, 7, 10, 13, 25, 33, 34, 47, 53, 73, 120, 128, 130, 131, 168, 172, 173, 174, 175
codon, 14, 25, 27, 29, 64, 124, 142, 152, 159
codon 157, 142
cognitive impairment, 155
colon, 4, 9, 10, 12, 14, 17, 35, 37, 44, 45, 50, 58, 60, 61, 68, 70, 74, 99, 107, 120, 130, 132, 139, 140, 141, 142, 143, 148, 153, 156
colon cancer, 35, 37, 45, 50, 60, 68, 70, 130, 142, 148, 153
colon polyps, 140, 153
colorectal cancer, 1, 5, 7, 8, 22, 31, 35, 36, 44, 45, 53, 72, 73, 94, 115, 120, 121, 124, 129, 133, 142, 147, 148, 153, 155, 168, 178, 181
common findings, 137
complications, 34
composition, 175
compounds, 19, 76, 173
conduction, 50
conjunctiva, 6, 140, 142
connective tissue, 49
consanguinity, 164
consensus, 63, 73

cooperation, 56
COPD, 122
COPS3, 103, 110
corepressor, 38, 176
correlation(s), 25, 39, 97, 108, 129, 137, 142, 143, 154, 160
cortex, 47
cortisol, 152
Cowden Syndrome, 140
CSF, 12, 30, 57, 59
CT, 111, 159
CTNNB1, 4, 17, 22, 60, 79, 85
cues, 38, 174
CV, 70, 110
cyclins, 14, 15
CYLD, 18, 72
cyst, 83, 89
cysteine, 12, 14
cytochrome, 118
cytokines, 57
cytoplasm, 29, 41, 174
cytosine, 37, 62, 168
cytoskeleton, 154

D

damages, 34
database, 112, 148, 165
DCUN1D1, 98, 103, 113
DDB2, 66, 67, 68
deacetylation, 175, 176
deaths, 76, 162
defects, 8, 16, 41, 52, 55, 135, 143, 158
deficiency(ies), 7, 8, 9, 24, 29, 66, 67, 139
degenerate, 18
degradation, 13, 15, 17, 22, 23, 71, 103, 110, 142
Delta, 40
dendritic cell, 123, 132
deposition, 156
deposits, 137
deregulation, 30, 177
derivatives, 21, 169
dermatosis, 18
detectable, 137, 150, 155, 160
detection, 80, 120, 139, 141, 147, 160
detoxification, 125
developmental disorder, 11
developmental process, 57, 61
diabetes, 28, 68
diagnostic criteria, 137, 150
dilation, 6
dimerization, 4, 23, 25, 37
diploid, 98

disability, 8
discrimination, 34
diseases, 4, 28, 39, 43, 46, 58, 62, 123, 128, 129, 131, 159
disequilibrium, 116, 119
disorder, 5, 6, 7, 10, 18, 20, 33, 34, 36, 39, 45, 49, 50, 52, 53, 54, 55, 57, 62, 65, 72, 86, 95, 138, 143, 146, 147, 148, 150, 155, 156, 159, 160, 161, 163, 182
dissociation, 47
distribution, 23, 28, 136, 168
diversity, 174
DNA damage, 5, 6, 9, 10, 21, 34, 37, 63, 66, 67, 74, 109, 124, 131, 145, 150, 164
DNA lesions, 21, 66
DNA Methylation, 168
DNA polymerase, 34, 67, 68, 164
DNA repair, 5, 6, 9, 17, 21, 34, 59, 63, 67, 68, 118, 123, 128, 169, 176
DNAs, 52
DNMT3A, 18, 19, 168, 179
domain structure, 175
dopamine, 43
double helix, 158
Drosophila, 45, 57, 59
drugs, 9, 97, 125, 177
duodenal polyps, 143
duodenum, 5, 151, 156
DYRK2, 98, 103, 111
Dyskeratosis Congenita, 141
dysplasia, 4, 23, 62, 65, 140

E

E2F3, 98, 103, 111
E-cadherin, 13, 14, 17, 59, 121
ectoderm, 46
EGFR, 19, 73, 98, 103, 110, 126
EIF5A2, 98, 103
electron, 24, 55
elongation, 20, 104, 123, 172
embryogenesis, x
embryonic stem cells, 132
EMS, 81, 87, 88, 89, 94, 181
encephalopathy, 24
encoding, ix, 3, 22, 27, 31, 41, 55, 59, 60, 76, 111, 123, 168, 172, 176
endocrine, 33, 47, 52, 140, 151, 152, 166
endocrine glands, 151, 152
endometrial carcinoma, 25, 35, 60
endometrial hyperplasia, 35
endonuclease, 34
endothelial cells, 118

energy, 24, 161
environment, 76, 174
environmental stresses, 32
enzymatic activity, 34, 44, 146
enzyme(s), 6, 18, 30, 37, 55, 72, 74, 123, 128, 169, 170, 171, 172, 173, 175
eosinophilia, 43, 83, 84, 86, 87, 91
EPC, 46
epidermoid cyst, 5, 143
epigenetic modification, x
epigenetic silencing, 35
epigenetics, 167
epilepsy, 65
epinephrine, 53
epithelia, 58
epithelial cells, 13, 53, 107, 120
epithelium, 13, 42, 64, 120, 143
ERBB2, 19, 20, 97, 98, 104
ERCC2, 66, 67, 68
erythropoietin, 30, 57
esophageal cancer, 98, 109, 123
esophagus, 15, 40, 64, 139, 142, 144, 156
estrogen, 27, 64, 102, 104, 110, 116, 117, 118, 145, 176
etiology, 37, 60, 64, 120, 122, 138, 160
EU, 130
euchromatin, 167, 172, 175
Europe, 60
evidence, 16, 40, 97, 122, 127, 133, 149, 153, 171, 176
excision, 34, 37, 66, 67, 72, 153, 164
exclusion, 35
execution, 12
exons, 14, 27, 35, 36, 48, 49, 53, 69, 150, 152, 160
exonuclease, 34, 68
exposure, 9, 10, 64, 125, 157
expressivity, 51
EXT1, 20, 21, 74, 147
EXT2, 20, 21, 74, 147
extracellular matrix, 161
EZH2, 46, 62, 173, 178, 179

F

FAM123B, 22
Familial Adenomatous Polyposis, 142, 153
families, ix, x, 9, 10, 13, 14, 17, 25, 34, 35, 36, 40, 44, 45, 51, 58, 63, 64, 73, 76, 115, 116, 140, 142, 143, 146, 147, 149, 150, 151, 155, 157, 158, 160, 161, 162, 170, 171, 173, 174, 175, 176
family history, 138, 146, 156, 163
family members, 16, 19, 23, 33, 45, 157, 174
FANCA, 21, 144

Fanconi Anemia pathway, 21, 51
fat, 28, 139
FBXW7, 22
FDA, 171
FDA approval, 171
femur, 147
fertilization, 138
FH, 24, 146
fibroblast growth factor, 23, 105, 116, 124
fibroids, 146
fibrosarcoma, 42, 76, 78, 92, 137
fibrosis, 142
fibrous tissue, 143
fidelity, 67, 119, 130
first degree relative, 35, 63
FLCN, 24, 25, 139
FLT3, 25, 26, 71, 91
formation, 20, 22, 29, 36, 38, 48, 53, 59, 69, 102, 105, 106, 109, 137, 161, 176
founder effect, 128
FOXL2, 26, 73
fragile site, 13
fragility, 11
frameshift mutation, ix, 22, 142, 154, 157, 159
France, 112
fumarate hydratase, 24
fusion, 2, 9, 16, 23, 40, 42, 43, 48, 54, 69, 70, 75, 76, 77, 80, 95, 171, 172, 173

G

G>T mutations, 37
gallbladder, 5, 10
ganglion, 53
gastrin, 151
gastroesophageal reflux, 64
gastrointestinal tract, 4, 31, 43, 49, 58, 62, 153, 156
GATA1, 26, 70, 170
GATA3, 27, 70, 126
GATA6, 99, 105, 111
GDP, 29, 41
gene amplification, ix, 4, 20, 44, 101, 102, 109, 111, 112, 113
gene expression, x, 18, 59, 97, 116, 119, 158, 167, 177
gene promoter, 170
gene regulation, 6
gene silencing, 119, 168, 171
genetic alteration, ix, 29, 55, 97, 173
genetic factors, 122
genetic mutations, ix
genetic predisposition, 120
genetic testing, 38, 95, 141

genetic traits, 135
genetics, 69, 71, 72, 115, 129, 144, 165, 166, 178
genitourinary tract, 163
genome, 1, 7, 9, 34, 66, 70, 73, 74, 97, 98, 115, 122, 130, 131, 151, 167, 168, 172, 176
genomic instability, 52
genomic stability, 9
genotype(ing), 25, 39, 53, 115, 116, 129, 137, 142, 154, 160
Germany, 155
germline mutations, 4, 5, 7, 9, 13, 25, 35, 37, 47, 55, 58, 61, 63, 69, 124, 137, 142, 146, 148, 150, 151
gingival, 141
gland, 17, 77, 81, 82, 85, 86, 90, 153, 176
glioblastoma, 19, 20, 31, 81, 98, 99, 106, 112
glioblastoma multiforme, 106
glioma, 49, 98, 99, 100, 102, 109, 111, 123, 128, 129
gluconeogenesis, 28
glucose, 3
glycogen, 28
GNAQ, 27, 73
GNAS, 27, 28, 74
goiter, 66
GPC5, 99, 105, 122
granules, 148
GRB7, 99, 104
growth, 2, 3, 6, 7, 13, 14, 19, 20, 23, 28, 29, 30, 31, 33, 38, 42, 44, 47, 50, 52, 56, 58, 64, 71, 73, 74, 76, 98, 99, 100, 103, 104, 106, 107, 108, 109, 118, 120, 122, 138, 139, 152, 156, 161, 171, 178
growth factor, 19, 20, 23, 42, 44, 50, 71, 76, 98, 99, 103, 106, 118
growth hormone, 28, 30, 152
guanine, 27, 37, 41
guidelines, 166

H

hair, 18, 24, 49, 52, 139, 158
hair follicle, 18, 24, 49, 139
half-life, 3
HBV, 60
HCC, 60, 177
HDAC, 171
HE, 111
hearing loss, 162
height, 159
hematopoietic stem cells, 143
hematopoietic system, 116
hepatitis, 17, 60
hepatocellular carcinoma, 17, 31, 60, 102, 110, 144, 160
hepatocytes, 28

Hereditary Breast/Ovarian Cancer, 144
Hereditary Diffuse Gastric Cancer, 146
hereditary hemorrhagic telangiectasia, 57
Hereditary Leiomyomatosis and Renal Cell Cancer, 146
Hereditary Multiple Exostosis, 147
Hereditary Nonpolyposis Colon Cancer, 147
Hereditary Papillary Renal Cell Carcinoma, 148
heritability, 115, 129
heterochromatin, 51, 167, 174, 175
heterogeneity, 25, 58, 77, 156, 165
histidine, 14, 172
histology, 112, 135
histone(s), x, 9, 33, 38, 40, 46, 51, 56, 67, 104, 167, 169, 170, 171, 172, 173, 174, 175, 176, 177, 178, 179
histone deacetylase, 9, 33, 170, 176, 178
history, 47, 71, 138, 146
HLA, 125, 126, 127
HM, 96, 178
homeostasis, 27
hormone(s), 27, 65
hotspots, 4, 10, 17, 23, 28, 29, 32, 39, 40, 41, 42, 43, 44, 48, 49, 50, 52, 54, 56, 57, 58, 59, 62, 63, 64, 140, 160
human, ix, 7, 23, 31, 40, 57, 59, 63, 64, 65, 70, 71, 72, 73, 75, 76, 77, 96, 97, 101, 103, 104, 108, 110, 112, 113, 115, 116, 128, 133, 170, 171, 173, 176, 177, 178, 179
human chorionic gonadotropin, 65
human development, 59
human genome, ix, 115, 116, 177
human skin, 23
Hunter, 132
hybrid, ix, 12, 75, 139, 173
hydrolysis, 27, 32
hypercalcemia, 34, 152
hyperinsulinemia, 34
hypermethylation, 168
hyperparathyroidism, 34, 52, 152, 153
hyperplasia, 31, 138, 150, 154
hypertelorism, 39, 50
hypertension, 53
hyperthyroidism, 66
hypertrophy, 143
hypoglycemia, 138
hypogonadism, 52
hypothesis, 77, 162
hypothyroidism, 66
hypoxia, 63, 120, 149, 161
hypoxia-inducible factor, 120, 161

I

ID, 70
ideal, 75
identification, ix, 115
identity, 42
IDH1, 29, 30, 70
IDH2, 29, 30, 70
idiopathic, 30, 62
idiopathic myelofibrosis, 30, 62
ileum, 156
imbalances, 112
imitation, 175
immune system, 136
immunodeficiency, 6, 136, 137, 155
immunoglobulin(s), 76, 80, 120
immunoglobulin superfamily, 120
immunohistochemistry, 145
imprinting, 138, 149
in vitro, 52, 138
in vivo, 36, 52, 139
incidence, 7, 9, 10, 36, 50, 51, 58, 77, 124, 137, 139, 140, 144, 149, 150, 151, 157, 160, 162, 164
individuals, 6, 12, 24, 39, 49, 60, 61, 120, 137, 139, 143, 144, 145, 146, 147, 151, 152, 153, 154, 156, 157, 160, 161, 162, 163, 164
indolent, 152
infancy, 8, 139, 158, 159, 160
infants, 69, 157
infection, 137
inflammation, 69, 172
infundibulum, 49
inheritance, ix, 50, 135, 136, 141
inhibition, 6, 11, 101, 112, 120, 171
inhibitor, 2, 15, 33, 57, 106, 112, 128
initiation, 5, 6, 66, 67, 98, 137, 168
inositol, 175
INS, 119
insertion, 7, 24, 34, 45, 46, 54, 66, 139, 151
institutions, x
insulin, 3, 28, 68, 118, 151
integrin(s), 59, 118
integrity, 10, 70, 104
interface, 50
interference, 106, 112
interferon (IFN), 57, 59, 123, 132
interferon-γ, 57, 123, 132
intestinal obstruction, 53
intestine, 53
intrauterine growth retardation, 12
intron, 26, 116, 159, 163
invasive cancer, 150
inversion, ix, 53, 96
iodine, 29
ionizing radiation, 6, 9, 136
iris, 39, 154
iron, 122
irradiation, 6, 145, 157
islands, 168

J

JAK2, 30, 72, 86, 88, 89, 127, 174, 175, 178
Japan, 162, 164
jejunum, 156
JUN, 33, 99, 105, 111

K

karyotype(ing), 16, 26, 77, 80, 155, 173
keratosis, 44
kidney(s), 8, 22, 24, 28, 56, 61, 65, 69, 116, 138, 148, 160, 163, 164
kidney tumors, 24, 148
kinase activity, 2, 20, 23, 30, 31, 42, 59, 71, 75, 76, 102
kinetochore, 11, 142
KIT, 31, 43, 71, 99, 105, 110
KLF6, 31, 72
KRAS, 9, 32, 37, 60
Krebs cycle, 55

L

landscape, 73
large intestine, 5, 6, 7, 8, 19, 20, 23, 27, 28, 32, 33, 36, 38, 40, 57, 61
larynx, 35, 139
lead, 4, 5, 9, 23, 25, 34, 38, 44, 48, 50, 72, 75, 120, 149, 162, 163
learning, 154
learning disabilities, 154
leiomyoma, 80, 87, 89, 91
leiomyomata, 146
lens, 38
lesions, 7, 8, 20, 24, 48, 50, 66, 135, 140, 141, 143, 146, 147, 150, 160, 162
leucine, 5
leukemia, 2, 6, 12, 26, 30, 39, 41, 43, 50, 54, 63, 64, 71, 73, 76, 83, 85, 86, 89, 90, 92, 94, 95, 98, 125, 137, 150, 154, 166, 170, 171, 174, 181
leukopenia, 159
lifetime, 10, 141, 142, 143, 148, 150, 157
ligament, 162
ligand, 3, 19, 23, 25, 40, 50

light, 67, 165
linear function, 96
lipolysis, 28
lipoma, 78, 85, 90, 91
liver, 5, 12, 17, 20, 26, 28, 31, 32, 52, 57, 60, 62, 64, 98, 107, 173, 177
liver cancer, 60, 177
localization, 41, 42
loci, 116, 118, 120, 122, 129, 130, 132, 147, 149, 163
locus, 10, 35, 40, 44, 45, 58, 98, 99, 100, 117, 120, 122, 124, 125, 128, 129, 130, 131, 132, 136, 147, 150, 155, 156, 163, 172, 176
lung cancer, 3, 4, 13, 19, 64, 95, 98, 101, 102, 103, 104, 106, 107, 109, 110, 111, 113, 114, 121, 122, 123, 128, 131, 132, 158, 182
lung disease, 65
Luo, 111, 113
luteinizing hormone, 65
lymph node, 31, 104, 108, 109, 113, 145, 177
lymphoid, 2, 6, 13, 17, 19, 23, 26, 30, 31, 36, 40, 41, 46, 54, 56, 58, 62, 63, 69, 85, 94, 139, 155, 173, 181
lymphoid tissue, 2, 6, 13, 19, 23, 26, 30, 31, 36, 40, 41, 46, 54, 56, 58, 62, 63, 69, 94, 173, 181
lymphoma, 3, 37, 41, 45, 58, 63, 80, 86, 90, 91, 92, 93, 94, 95, 96, 100, 108, 118, 126, 132, 137, 150, 155, 166, 171, 173, 174, 181, 182
lysine, 46, 56, 169, 170, 171, 172, 173, 174, 179

M

machinery, 56, 66
macroglossia, 138
macrosomia, 138
majority, ix, 4, 20, 25, 29, 32, 33, 38, 49, 50, 58, 116, 118, 129, 135, 137, 140, 142, 145, 150, 151, 157
malignancy, 4, 12, 36, 49, 55, 63, 69, 145, 148, 155, 157, 158, 176
malignant cells, 168, 169
malignant melanoma, 8, 14, 15, 50, 64, 92, 101, 107, 164
malignant mesothelioma, 6, 70
malignant tumors, ix, 5, 36, 45, 58, 120, 151, 152, 157
mammalian cells, 59
management, 39, 96, 165
mantle, 80, 91
MAP3K1, 32, 33, 116, 117, 118
MAP3K13, 33
MAP3K5, 99, 105, 110
mapping, 97, 105, 112

Marc Lacroix, iii, x
mass, 18, 37, 53
mast cells, 62
matrix, 55, 59, 176
MB, 70, 78, 111, 112
MDM2, 99, 103, 106, 112
MDM4, 99, 106
MED29, 99, 106
median, 4, 67, 68, 137, 147, 163, 164
medical, 12, 165
medicine, 131
medulla, 43, 53, 55
medulloblastoma, 7, 11, 22, 59, 99, 104, 107, 137, 146, 155, 158, 173
MEK, 8
melanin, 156
melanoma, 6, 8, 14, 15, 27, 50, 67, 70, 73, 98, 99, 102, 106, 113, 116, 122, 128, 159, 162, 164, 174
mellitus, 28
MEN1, 33, 34, 151, 152
meninges, 39
meningioma, 7, 31, 39, 49, 92, 137, 158
mental retardation, 29, 39, 65, 69, 163
mesentery, 5, 48
mesoderm, 159
mesothelioma, 39
MET, 99, 106, 108, 112, 113, 148, 149
meta-analysis, 127, 132
metabolic pathways, 24
metabolism, 2, 3, 24, 63, 100, 119, 123, 125, 128, 146, 156, 161, 165
metal ion, 171
metastasis, 13, 102, 104, 108, 109, 110, 111, 113, 120, 121, 132, 149, 176, 177
metastatic disease, 152
methyl groups, 18
methylation, x, 18, 25, 34, 46, 56, 128, 138, 149, 167, 168, 169, 171, 172, 174, 177
Mg^{2+}, 99
mice, 32, 110, 120
microcephaly, 12, 155, 161
migration, 4, 19, 65, 101, 102, 111
MITF, 99, 106
mitochondria, 29
mitogen(s), 19, 42, 105, 117, 120
mitosis, x
MLH1, 7, 9, 34, 35, 36, 44, 45, 120, 145, 148
modelling, 177
models, 170, 176
modifications, x, 167, 169, 172, 173, 175, 178, 179
modules, 179
mole, 15
molecules, 9, 13, 24, 27, 33, 44, 50, 123, 172

morbidity, 39, 143, 154
morphology, 62
mortality, 39, 137, 143
mosaic, 11, 154, 157, 165
motif, 5, 12, 22, 41, 49, 119, 171
MPL, 36, 70
mRNA, 3, 104, 108, 132, 145
MSH2, 7, 9, 34, 35, 36, 44, 45, 120, 145, 148
MSH6, 7, 9, 34, 35, 36, 115, 120, 148
MTDH, 99, 107, 111
mucosa, 142, 146, 173
Multiple Endocrine Neoplasia Type 1, 151
Multiple Endocrine Neoplasia Type 2A, 2B, 152
multiple myeloma, 23, 98, 102
multiple primary tumors, 164
muscles, 5
musculoskeletal, 29
mutagenesis, 165
mutant, 1, 25, 64, 70, 71, 132, 155, 179
mutation rate, 37, 39, 142
MUTYH, 37, 74, 153
MYC, 37, 38, 70, 72, 84, 85, 88, 89, 98, 99, 107, 110, 111, 124, 127, 129, 132, 142, 170, 176
MYCL1, 99, 107
MYCN, 97, 99, 107, 112
myelin, 38
myelodysplasia, 56, 142, 159
myelodysplastic syndromes, 12, 25, 72, 178, 179
myelofibrosis, 62
myeloproliferative disorders, 30, 62
MYH-Associated Polyposis, 153
myocardial infarction, 68
myopathy, 29

N

NAD, 171
NADH, 24
nasopharyngeal carcinoma, 31, 128
NCOA3, 89, 99, 107, 108, 170
NCOR1, 38
negativity, 104
neoplasm, 43, 53, 86, 87, 90, 91, 138, 164
nephropathy, 69, 163
nerve, 38, 39, 61, 154
nervous system, 94, 107, 154, 164, 181
neural system, 15
neuroblastoma, 4, 43, 50, 70, 97, 98, 99, 107, 138
Neurofibromatosis Type 1, 153
Neurofibromatosis Type 2, 154
neurons, 65
neurotransmitter(s), 27, 43
neurotrophic factors, 52

nevoid basal cell carcinoma syndrome, 48
nevus, 9, 15, 86
next generation, 178
NF1, 38, 39, 74, 153, 154
NF2, 38, 39, 74, 154, 155
Nijmegen Breakage Syndrome, 155
nitrogen, 173
NKX2-1, 99, 101, 127
nodules, 39, 154, 161
nonsense mutation, 14, 17, 38, 53, 66, 160
norepinephrine, 53
normal aging, 162
normal development, 68
North America, 153
NOTCH1, 40, 72, 88
NPM1, 4, 40, 41, 71, 84, 85, 87
NRAS, 8, 14, 41
NTRK3, 41, 42, 76, 78, 79, 92, 96
nuclear receptors, 38
nucleic acid, 7, 40
nucleosome, 74, 167, 169, 175, 176, 178, 179
nucleotides, 59, 67, 176
nucleus, 17, 43, 130, 142, 174, 177
null, 47
nutrient, 58

O

obesity, 166
ocular hypertelorism, 50
oesophageal, 131
oligodendrocytes, 38
oncogenes, 1, 76, 129, 170, 171
oncogenesis, 97, 169, 176, 177
oncoproteins, 170
opportunities, 72
optic nerve, 154
oral cavity, 14
organ(s), 9, 10, 49, 51, 58, 65, 93, 135, 136, 140, 145, 160, 161
osteodystrophy, 28
osteogenic sarcoma, 52, 159
osteoporosis, 68
ovarian cancer, 3, 9, 10, 14, 20, 26, 37, 51, 60, 98, 100, 103, 108, 111, 112, 118, 129, 130, 135, 144, 145, 165
ovarian tumor, 3, 10, 15, 47, 53, 128, 133, 145, 151
ovaries, 9, 10, 48, 49, 51, 58
overlap, 49, 69
oxidation, 55, 169, 179
oxidative damage, 29
oxidative stress, 30

P

p53, 5, 17, 25, 40, 56, 58, 63, 68, 71, 99, 103, 106, 109, 132, 136, 150, 151, 170
PAK1, 99, 108, 113
palate, 127
PALB2, 11, 21, 22, 42, 73, 115, 116, 144
pancreas, 5, 10, 15, 17, 20, 32, 33, 40, 60, 61, 91, 98, 100, 101, 105, 116, 128, 151, 156
pancreatic cancer, 15, 60, 101, 105, 106, 111, 140, 143, 145
pancreatic insufficiency, 159
parathyroid, 25, 28, 33, 34, 150
parathyroid hormone, 34
parents, 136
pathogenesis, 13, 72, 74, 95, 128, 165
pathways, 9, 18, 19, 28, 32, 42, 47, 72, 73, 101, 110, 116, 168, 174, 177
PAX9, 99, 101, 111
PCM, 80
PCR, 80
PDGFRA, 31, 42, 43, 81, 84, 86
pediatrician, 166
pelvis, 154, 156
penetrance, ix, 5, 10, 17, 36, 39, 51, 115, 118, 120, 122, 130, 139, 143, 144, 147, 148, 151, 153, 156, 157, 158, 161, 163
penis, 49, 140
peptic ulcer disease, 34
peptidase, 118
peptide, 152
peripheral blood, 62
peripheral nervous system, 39
peritoneum, 145
permit, 150
peroxide, 33
Peutz–Jeghers Syndrome, 156
pharynx, 10
phenotype(s), 16, 19, 22, 25, 35, 36, 39, 43, 44, 45, 49, 53, 74, 101, 108, 118, 128, 136, 137, 138, 142, 143, 145, 154, 160, 163, 176
pheochromocytoma, 52, 53, 71, 165
Philadelphia, 30, 75
phosphate, 174
phosphorylation, 2, 6, 8, 15, 23, 25, 30, 32, 47, 98, 111, 136, 169, 172, 174
PHOX2B, 1, 43, 70
physicians, 138
PI3K, 42, 44, 49, 72, 141
pigmentation, 39, 47, 52, 140
PIK3CA, 44, 60, 73, 99, 108, 111
pituitary tumors, 28
plasma membrane, 22, 29, 41

playing, 2
pleura, 6, 15, 39, 128
plexus, 64, 158
ploidy, 97
PM, 112
PMS1, 34, 44, 148
PMS2, 34, 45, 120, 148
pneumothorax, 138
point mutation, ix, 3, 4, 10, 17, 20, 22, 23, 25, 28, 29, 37, 38, 39, 40, 42, 50, 52, 54, 56, 58, 62, 65, 142, 157, 160, 163, 164
polarity, 156
POLH, 66, 67, 68
polyamine, 128
Polycomb group (PcG) proteins, 45
polycomb group proteins, 73
polycomb repressive complex, 45, 176, 178
polycystic kidney disease, 160
polycythemia vera, 30, 62
polydactyly, 48
polymer, 96
polymerase, 9, 34, 66, 118
polymerization, 101
polymorphism(s), ix, 11, 116, 117, 121, 123, 127, 132, 133, 145
polyostotic fibrous dysplasia, 28
polypeptide(s), 42, 99, 100, 118
Polyposis, Familial Juvenile, 156
polyp(s), 4, 8, 35, 45, 58, 59, 120, 141, 142, 143, 153, 154, 156, 157
population, ix, 77, 115, 116, 118, 136, 139, 141, 142, 143, 144, 149, 150, 151, 152, 153, 155, 156, 157, 163, 164
PPM1D, 99, 109, 112
PPP2R1A, 47, 60, 72
precursor cells, 62, 160
premature death, 65
preparation, 158
preservation, 26
primary hyperparathyroidism, 34
primary tumor, 106, 112, 135, 157, 173, 177
prior knowledge, 116
PRKAR1A, 47, 48, 54, 70, 80, 90, 93, 140
PRKCI, 99, 108, 113
probability, 103
probands, 150
progenitor cells, 25
progesterone, 110, 116, 145
prognosis, 16, 59, 64, 80, 101, 104, 106, 107, 111, 129, 149, 169, 172, 173
prolactin, 30
proliferation, 2, 3, 4, 16, 17, 19, 25, 31, 33, 37, 38, 40, 41, 44, 48, 55, 59, 62, 65, 100, 103, 104, 105,

Index

112, 116, 121, 122, 128, 131, 149, 151, 152, 154, 160, 166, 176
proline, 169
promoter, 25, 27, 67, 120, 124, 128, 141, 157, 168
prophylactic, 146
prostate cancer, 3, 7, 9, 20, 31, 72, 77, 93, 99, 101, 110, 115, 119, 120, 129, 130, 131, 133, 145, 173
proteasome, 110, 122
protection, 29, 73, 121
protein design, 154, 155
protein family, 14, 22
protein kinase C, 112
protein kinases, 2, 3, 58, 174, 175
proteins, ix, 2, 4, 5, 6, 7, 13, 14, 19, 20, 21, 22, 24, 25, 29, 30, 32, 33, 37, 43, 45, 46, 47, 48, 49, 54, 56, 57, 62, 67, 68, 71, 73, 75, 76, 97, 103, 109, 128, 145, 151, 157, 167, 168, 169, 170, 171, 172, 174
proto-oncogene, 1, 77, 99, 107, 148
pseudohypoparathyroidism, 28
PTEN, 8, 44, 49, 50, 60, 63, 73, 116, 141, 145, 156, 170
PTPN11, 50
pulmonary stenosis, 39
pulmonic stenosis, 50
pyrimidine, 67

R

RAB25, 99, 108, 110
RAD51C, 9, 10, 21, 51, 73, 116, 144
radiation, 128, 131, 136, 155, 157
rash, 141, 158
RASSF1, 131
RB1, 51, 52, 70, 122, 157, 158
RE, 165
reactive oxygen, 153
reading, 128, 172
receptors, 12, 13, 27, 30, 36, 59, 71, 145
reciprocal translocation, 81
recognition, 13, 66, 174
recombination, 7, 9, 10, 11, 30, 51, 52, 116, 162, 174
recommendations, 165
recruiting, 176
rectum, 4, 142, 156
recurrence, 113
red blood cells, 26
regression, 106
relatives, 5, 35, 115, 136, 156
relaxation, 102
relaxation process, 102
relevance, 178
remodelling, 128

renal cell carcinoma, 6, 24, 61, 71, 72, 76, 83, 93, 139, 147, 149, 161, 166
renal failure, 69, 163
repair, 6, 8, 9, 11, 21, 34, 36, 37, 42, 44, 45, 48, 51, 66, 67, 68, 71, 72, 102, 120, 145, 148, 150, 153, 155, 162, 164, 166
replication, x, 7, 21, 34, 48, 51, 66, 67, 68, 71, 102, 136, 158, 162, 164, 168
repression, 26, 45, 51, 125, 128, 169, 172, 176
repressor, 38, 120, 174, 177
RES, 171, 176
resection, 151
residues, 50, 168, 169, 171, 172, 174, 175
resistance, 36, 66, 108, 110, 111, 112
resolution, 21, 110, 113, 177
response, 10, 16, 32, 43, 57, 67, 73, 74, 107, 113, 117, 123, 124, 132, 136, 149, 164, 171
RET, 1, 48, 52, 53, 54, 72, 76, 80, 82, 83, 87, 88, 90, 96, 152, 172, 178
retardation, 6, 50, 161
reticulum, 20
retina, 51, 106, 157
retinoblastoma, 14, 51, 99, 106, 112, 157
retroviruses, 28
reverse transcriptase, 96, 127, 132, 141
Rhabdoid Tumor Predisposition Syndrome, 158
ribosome, 40, 159
risk factors, 123, 130
risks, 10, 143, 145, 148, 151, 153, 156, 157, 159
RNA, 9, 18, 56, 66, 106, 112, 118, 128, 130, 141, 167, 176
RNA splicing, 56
RNAs, 168, 176, 179
Rothmund–Thomson Syndrome, 158
routes, 110
RPS6KB1, 100, 109
RTS, 52, 158, 159
RUNX1, 54, 55, 62, 72, 76, 81, 82, 83, 84, 85, 86, 87, 88, 89, 91, 92, 93, 94, 143, 169

S

salivary gland(s), 17, 20, 29, 31, 49, 76, 87, 88, 89
SAS, 109, 112
scent, 18
sclera, 140
sclerosis, 58, 64, 65, 69, 72, 95, 152, 160, 163, 166, 181
SDHA, 55, 56, 149
SDHAF2, 55, 149
SDHB, 55, 56, 149
SDHC, 55, 56, 149
SDHD, 55, 56, 149, 150

sebaceous cyst, 5, 36, 45
secrete, 18, 151, 152
secretion, 8, 53
segregation, 11, 52
senescence, 63, 121, 123
sensitivity, 65, 102, 111, 128, 131, 143, 145, 155, 164, 177
sensors, 9
sequencing, 131, 141, 160
serine, 2, 3, 5, 7, 8, 14, 32, 33, 47, 49, 58, 77, 100, 112, 136, 174, 175
serotonin, 151
serum, 43
sex, 45, 135, 156, 163
sex reversal, 163
shape, 26, 38, 155
shelter, 142
showing, 12, 39, 173
Shwachman-Bodian-Diamond Syndrome, 159
sibling, 157
side chain, 172
signal peptide, 76
signal transduction, 19, 23, 28, 30, 32, 38, 56, 109, 174
signaling pathway, 13, 18, 19, 21, 22, 25, 31, 38, 49, 55, 57, 58, 59, 73, 77, 101, 105, 108, 120, 122, 154, 156
signalling, 71, 110, 133
signals, 27, 104, 106
signs, 49, 62, 154
Simpson–Golabi–Behmel Syndrome, 159
single-nucleotide polymorphism, 115, 118
siRNA, 100, 105
skin, 5, 7, 15, 18, 24, 29, 31, 35, 39, 41, 42, 44, 47, 48, 49, 56, 57, 58, 61, 62, 64, 65, 67, 91, 124, 128, 130, 136, 137, 139, 140, 141, 150, 153, 156, 159, 160, 164
skin cancer, 64, 67, 137, 150
SKP2,, 114
SMAD4, 56, 57, 101, 121, 156, 157
small intestine, 32, 35, 42, 86, 154, 156
smoking, 122, 123, 158
smooth muscle, 8, 65
smooth muscle cells, 65
SNP, 116, 117, 118, 119, 120, 121, 122, 123, 124, 125, 126, 127, 129, 132
SOCS1, 57, 58
sodium, 65, 118
soft tissue tumors, 106
solid tumors, 22, 50, 71, 76, 77, 103, 128, 143, 170
somatic alterations, 60
somatic cell, 107

somatic mutations, 3, 4, 5, 14, 16, 21, 24, 25, 26, 27, 31, 36, 39, 40, 46, 48, 49, 50, 59, 61, 158, 171, 175
species, 122, 153
speculation, 77
spina bifida, 48
spinal cord tumor, 155
spinal tumor, 39
spindle, 11, 125, 159, 161
spleen, 31, 62
spontaneous pneumothorax, 24
squamous cell, 144,
squamous cell carcinoma, 4, 22, 29, 37, 48, 64, 93, 98, 99, 100, 102, 103, 104, 108, 109, 111, 112, 113, 142, 159, 164, 172, 173
SS, 71, 110, 178
SSI, 57
stability, 11, 54, 55, 125, 151
stabilization, 142
STARD3, 100, 104
state(s), 13, 15, 27, 107, 169, 172, 174
stem cells, 119
stenosis, 142
stimulation, 57, 149
STK11, 58, 59, 116, 145, 156
stomach, 5, 6, 8, 10, 20, 23, 35, 36, 39, 42, 44, 52, 107, 141, 151, 156, 157, 164
storage, 28
strabismus, 51
stratification, 96
stress, 2, 109, 128
stress response, 2, 109
stroma, 8, 53
structural changes, 65
structural protein, 26
structure, x, 6, 51, 67, 149, 158, 167, 169, 171, 174, 175
style, 123
subgroups, 11, 14, 35, 178
substitution(s), 2, 3, 6, 8, 10, 12, 13, 15, 18, 19, 20, 22, 23, 26, 27, 28, 29, 31, 32, 33, 35, 36, 37, 38, 39, 40, 41, 42, 43, 44, 46, 48, 49, 50, 51, 56, 57, 59, 60, 61, 68, 69, 142, 173, 175
substrate(s), 2, 3, 6, 31
sucrose, 175
SUFU, 59, 70
Sun, 178
suppression, 42, 71, 109, 122, 152, 177
surface layer, 53
surveillance, 9, 34
survival, 2, 3, 25, 27, 32, 38, 44, 47, 49, 68, 73, 100, 102, 104, 106, 107, 109, 110, 111, 113, 132, 166, 168

Index

susceptibility, ix, 9, 10, 11, 35, 42, 43, 44, 45, 69, 72, 73, 115, 116, 118, 122, 123, 127, 128, 129, 130, 131, 132, 133, 135, 143, 145, 148, 149, 158
sweat, 18
SWI/SNF, 59, 60, 61, 74, 158, 175, 176, 179
sympathetic nervous system, 43
symptoms, 39, 65, 154, 156, 162
synthesis, 6, 9, 65, 67
systemic mastocytosis, 62

T

T cell, 17, 32, 40, 76, 95, 171, 178, 182
target, 17, 24, 26, 37, 47, 58, 63, 64, 71, 106, 107, 108, 110, 111, 112, 114, 129, 142, 171, 172, 174, 177, 178
TBX3, 61, 72
TCR, 76
techniques, 77, 141
technological advances, 1
technologies, 115
teeth, 143
telangiectasia, 6, 7, 52, 135, 137
telomere, 6, 123, 128, 139, 142
telomere shortening, 142
tendon sheath, 83
testicle, 164
testicular cancer, 105
testing, 138, 150, 165
testis, 26, 28, 31, 32, 41, 49, 52, 116, 156
TET2, 62, 69, 119, 169
TGF, 7, 24, 33, 56, 101, 120
therapeutic agents, 106
therapeutic targets, 178
therapeutics, 80
therapy, 71, 72, 96, 101, 111, 123, 132
threonine, 2, 3, 5, 7, 8, 14, 32, 33, 47, 49, 58, 112, 136, 174, 175
thrombopoietin, 36, 70
thymoma, 98
thymus, 33, 52, 151
thyroglobulin, 65
thyroid, 1, 3, 5, 8, 9, 14, 19, 23, 28, 29, 39, 41, 47, 48, 49, 52, 53, 56, 57, 65, 66, 76, 82, 83, 84, 87, 88, 90, 140, 141, 143, 150, 152, 160, 162, 166, 172, 178
thyroid cancer, 1, 9, 29, 49, 52, 76, 141, 143, 152, 160, 166
thyroid stimulating hormone, 65
tinnitus, 162
tissue, 12, 23, 28, 31, 33, 42, 50, 53, 61, 63, 65, 77, 78, 79, 80, 85, 90, 96, 100, 120, 129, 133, 137, 139, 141, 151, 162, 176, 177

TNF, 62
tobacco smoke, 64, 164
toddlers, 157
TP53, 1, 16, 40, 60, 62, 63, 64, 101, 110, 116, 122, 125, 145, 150
trafficking, 44, 108
transcription, x, 2, 4, 9, 12, 16, 17, 21, 22, 26, 27, 33, 37, 38, 43, 46, 51, 54, 56, 57, 61, 66, 67, 68, 76, 98, 99, 101, 102, 103, 105, 107, 113, 116, 117, 119, 129, 142, 143, 151, 161, 169, 170, 174, 175, 176, 177, 178
transcription factors, 2, 17, 26, 27, 38, 61, 76, 101, 169, 170, 174, 176, 177
transcripts, ix, 27, 40, 173
transducer, 174
transformation, 20, 37, 41, 50, 58, 63, 75, 77, 96, 105, 147, 149, 159, 162, 168, 170, 176
transforming growth factor, 19, 118
transitional cell carcinoma, 48
translation, 6, 13, 16, 98, 104
translocation, ix, 2, 16, 23, 26, 37, 40, 41, 42, 48, 53, 54, 69, 75, 77, 104, 169, 172
transmembrane glycoprotein, 20
transmission, 138
transport, 55
transversion mutation, 8
treatment, 54, 69, 94, 95, 145, 165, 166, 171, 181, 182
tricarboxylic acid cycle, 24, 146
triggers, 149, 174
trisomy, 172
tryptophan, 41, 100
TSC1, 64, 65, 160
TSC2, 64, 65, 160
TSH, 65, 66, 71
TSHR, 65, 66
TSPAN31, 100, 109
Tuberous Sclerosis Complex, 160
tumor cells, 105
tumor development, 55, 71, 112, 124, 130
tumor growth, 142, 149
tumor necrosis factor, 62, 177
tumor progression, 103, 107
tumorigenesis, 9, 48, 58, 77, 112, 120, 128, 132, 137, 178
tumour suppressor genes, 71
tumours, 71, 110, 111, 112
tyrosine, 2, 3, 4, 13, 19, 20, 23, 25, 30, 31, 36, 41, 42, 43, 49, 50, 52, 53, 57, 71, 72, 75, 76, 96, 98, 103, 106, 110, 111, 112, 116, 118, 173, 174, 175, 178
Tyrosine, 3, 25, 41, 50, 100

U

ubiquitin, 17, 21, 22, 71, 74, 99, 100, 169
ubiquitin-proteasome system, 17
UES, 80
umbilical cord, 26
United States, 60, 145, 155, 164
upper respiratory tract, 139
ureters, 156
urethra, 142
urinary tract, 3, 5, 15, 29, 32, 39, 44, 52, 53, 65, 128, 148
urine, 133
uterine cancer, 137
uterus, 10, 35, 58, 156, 164
UV, 10, 64, 67, 164
UV light, 10

V

valine, 142
variations, 42
Variegated Aneuploidy, Mosaic, 161
vertigo, 162
vesicle, 108
vestibular schwannoma, 39, 40, 154, 155
viral infection, 63
vision, 154
Von Hippel–Lindau Syndrome, 161
vulva, 17, 49, 140

W

WD, 22
web, 150
Werner Syndrome, 68, 139, 162, 165
WHSC1L1, 88, 100, 104
wild type, 24, 109
Wilms Tumor, Familial, 163
Wnt signaling, 22, 58
worldwide, 116, 136, 149
wound healing, 148
WRN, 68, 123, 139, 162
WT1, 22, 68, 69, 78, 91, 163

X

xenografts, 106
Xeroderma Pigmentosum, 66, 67, 164, 165
XPA, 66, 67, 68
XPC, 66, 67, 68

Y

yeast, 118
yield, 38
young people, 93
young women, 65
YWHAB, 100, 107, 109
YWHAQ, 100, 109
YWHAZ, 100, 109

Z

zinc, 69, 111, 118, 163, 171
ZNF217, 100, 107
ZNF639, 100, 109
Zollinger-Ellison syndrome, 34